101
WAYS TO WORK OUT
WITH WEIGHTS

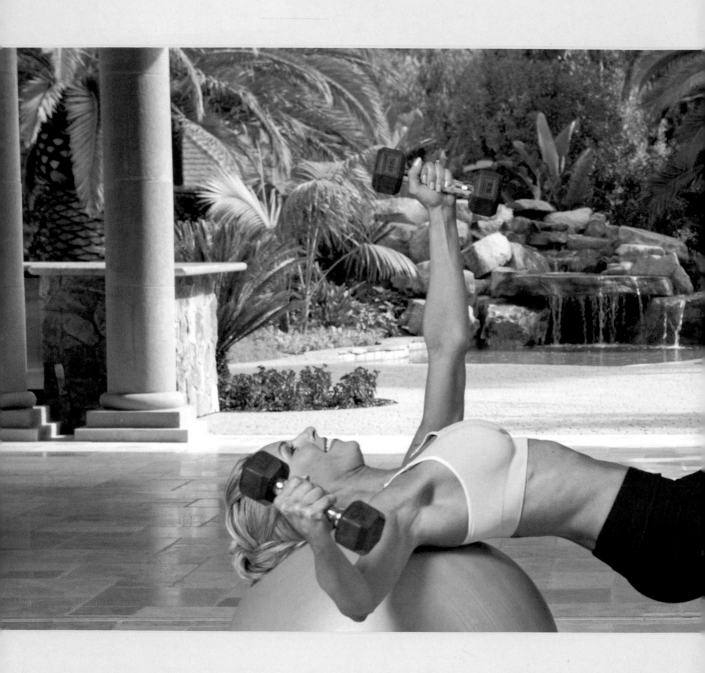

101
WAYS TO WORK OUT
WITH WEIGHTS

Effective Exercises to Sculpt Your Body and Burn Fat!

CINDY WHITMARSH

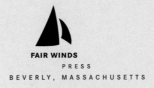

FAIR WINDS
PRESS
BEVERLY, MASSACHUSETTS

Text © 2006 by Cindy Whitmarsh
First published in the USA in 2006 by
Fair Winds Press, a member of
Quayside Publishing Group
100 Cummings Center
Suite 406-L
Beverly, MA 01915-6101

10 09   7 8 9

ISBN - 13: 978-1-59233-216-8
ISBN - 10: 1-59233-216-1

Library of Congress Cataloging-in-Publication Data available

Cover design by Laura Herrmann Design
Book layout by Leslie Haimes
Photography by Allan Penn
Printed and bound in Singapore

The information in this book is for educational purposes only. It is not
intended to replace the advice of a physician or medical practitioner. Please
see your health care provider before beginning any new health program.

I would like to dedicate this book to my parents, Ken and Mona.
Being a mommy has opened my eyes to the responsibility and selflessness
of a parent's love for their children.
I thank you for being the role models that every child should have,
and the inspiration that has helped mold me into the person I am today!

Contents

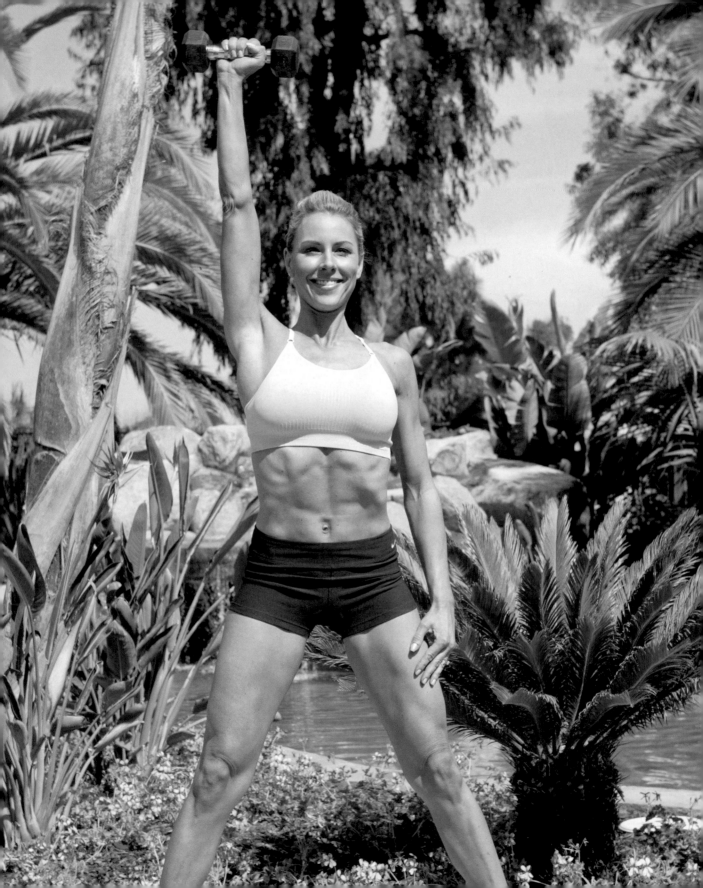

Testimonials

I first met Cindy four years ago at a beach volleyball tournament with her husband, Mike Whitmarsh. I was extremely impressed by her physique and overall fitness level, and as soon as I found out about her nutrition and personal training background, I started talking to her about the importance of effective weight training and a solid nutrition plan.

Being a professional beach volleyball player, I need to be lean and powerful, and Cindy's methods help me maintain my physique without impacting my energy level or performance. Cindy has been an inspiration to many of us in the pro beach volleyball circuit, and I've been witness to the total body transformation of countless friends through Cindy's dynamic workout routines and her Ultrafit Nutrition Program. In fact, my husband Casey and I take her book *Ultrafit* with us on tour to help us train and stay on top of our game. Cindy is a walking testimonial to the power of a lifestyle dedicated to health and fitness.

—Kerri Walsh
Beach Volleyball Olympic Gold Medalist

Knowing of her reputation for training athletes, I called Cindy during my last pregnancy to see if she would be willing to take me on as a client post-pregnancy. I've played professional beach volleyball for over 10 years with her husband Mike, and since meeting Cindy, he has been in the best shape of his life. Cindy's workouts really focus on the importance of core training, and getting my core strength back was imperative for me to compete professionally again after having my baby. I implemented Cindy's Ultrafit Nutrition Program as well as her high-intensity cross-training workouts and lost 25 pounds, 10 percent body fat, and a total of over 30 inches. Now I'm in the best shape of my life. Not only is it easier for me to keep up with my children, I'm ready to hit the beach again! I feel faster, stronger, and more confident than I've ever been. Thanks so much Cindy, you are the best!"

—Barbra Fontana,
Pro Beach Volleyball Player

66 Cindy's workouts are amazing...effective, innovative, and challenging enough to make you feel like you accomplished something but not too hard where you feel inept.

Her variety of workouts makes me look forward to exercising. I noticed an incredible difference working with Cindy in just a few weeks. Cindy's training has allowed me to stay competitive; play softball, golf, and over-the-line softball; and catch major league fly balls!

Cindy knows how to maximize the cardiovascular system while focusing on every muscle in your body! With my incredibly busy schedule, I am able to do Cindy's workouts and maintain muscle tone."

—Nina Detrow,
San Diego Padres Ball Girl
and Four-Time Over-the-Line Beach Softball World Champion

66 Cindy Whitmarsh saved me from years of destruction—it's a story that many people can probably relate to. I've been in the fitness industry for over 10 years, as a fitness competitor and fitness instructor. I studied nutrition in college, so I thought I was living a pretty healthy lifestyle. By the time I met Cindy, I was convinced I could never eat another carbohydrate again. I knew how to go to extremes for competitions, but I couldn't find the right balance that would allow me to maintain the physique I desired. I fell into a downward spiral of fad diet after diet, and my weight constantly fluctuated. I was miserable and I just couldn't figure it out. After countless discussions with Cindy (and several heated debates!), I finally began to understand the Ultrafit philosophy, especially when my body started looking the way I'd wanted it to look for so long! Cindy taught me that I didn't need to work out as hard or as often if I was eating correctly and if my workouts were efficient. Now, as the mother of twins and *still* a fitness instructor, I am also a nutrition consultant for Ultrafit and lead the six-week fitness challenges, and postpartum challenges. I now have the ability to help people like myself who are so lost with all the fad diets and nutrition information out there and just need a simple road map to get them back to being healthy. I will always thank Cindy for giving me my life back!"

—Jessica Janc, Encinitas, CA

66 Cindy's workout programs are the only things that have worked for me. I just had my fourth baby, and I am more fit now than I have ever been! The workouts are totally challenging but not so difficult that you feel defeated. I never thought that after four babies, I could ever feel as good as I do now. Cindy's dynamic workouts kicked my butt into shape! Everyone should try them!"

—Nicole Senalik,
mother of four, San Diego, CA

66 Cindy's workouts are always fun and interesting while giving you a killer body. She believes in multitasking to the hilt, and I love it! Every workout is intense and thorough, and I like the feeling that I'm not wasting any time. In addition, seeing Cindy's own body transformation in the past years has been very inspirational. It's hard to believe she has had two kids! One of the most important things I've learned after following Cindy's Ultrafit Fitness and Nutrition Programs is that exercise is vital, but nutrition is up to 70 percent of it. I now realize that you can exercise your heart out, but if you do not eat correctly, you can only get so far. Cindy has taught us not to starve ourselves. Instead, we have learned to eat healthy portions and add more protein to our diets. I struggled my whole life before Ultrafit, and now that I have reached my own level of Ultrafitness, I will be this way forever thanks to Cindy! It has also been wonderful to see the transformation in the many individuals who follow Cindy's program. Thanks, Cindy, for changing my life!"

—Moody Cabanillas, San Diego, CA

66 I came to see Cindy because my husband and friends were having a competition to see who could get in the best shape in six weeks. We all tried something different. Their plans included drastic dieting and extreme workout plans. I followed the Ultrafit Program, and not only did I win our little competition, but in the end I found a newer, more favorable lifestyle. I ate more than everyone else and worked out for less time, but with more intensity, and my results were dramatic! But the most amazing part was that I found a routine that fit right into my everyday life. It's not a crazy deprivation diet or extreme program that's impossible to maintain. The Ultrafit Program is the only way a plan is going to work for the long run."

—Corinne McKendrick, San Diego, CA

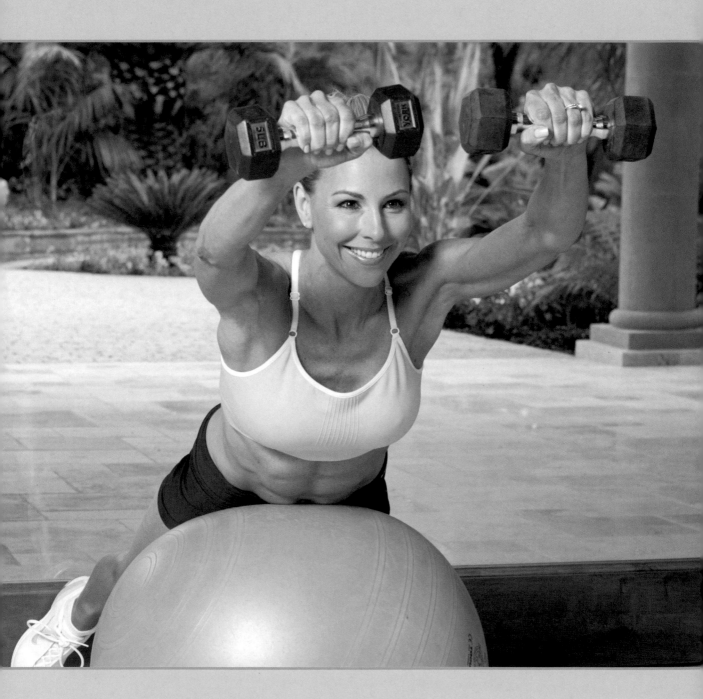

Introduction

What's the quickest path to the "perfect" body?

Hmmm…countless fitness magazines feature quick and easy routines and nutritional advice every month. I read through them, just like you do. I try to learn something new that might make life a little easier, just like you do. And I've still had to learn through success and failure, just like you have. It used to be that people thought they had to starve themselves and spend hours in the gym, but that's just not true. I know this because I live it on a daily basis. Life does not need to revolve around your cardio routine and the number of carbs you've eaten for the day! It just doesn't need to be so difficult!

Through diligence and hard work, I've been blessed with a body that's very lean and sculpted. I've worked at adopting a lifestyle and fitness regimen to create this body, and to maintain my accomplishments without living a life that feels stressed and deprived. I definitely experienced challenges within my own body-sculpting and weight-loss efforts, but through some serious trial and error, I learned that doing just cardio or dieting alone will never truly change a person's body. The ultimate key is time management—you have to use your time effectively and keep it interesting.

The number one question that people ask me is in regard to my cardio routine. Do I run? Do I bike? Which machines do I use in the gym? How long? How often? Okay, *listen up!* The *only way* to develop a lean, sculpted, and defined body is to incorporate weight training and to *stop* being so fixated on cardio! The truth is you need to have a balance of sensible nutrition, regular cardio, and effective weight training that challenges your body in order to affect your basal metabolic rate (the rate at which your body burns calories). Simply put, lean muscle burns more calories at rest than fat does. By changing your body composition through losing body fat and gaining lean muscle, you'll burn more calories even when you sleep! Isn't that the goal? To make our bodies more efficient so we don't have to work so hard? My previous book, *Ultrafit: Challenging Workouts, Amazing Results*, encompassed all three essential elements of my training philosophy—core training, interval training, and cross-training—and provided readers with a complete six-week guide to accomplishing various levels of "ultra"-fitness. If you already have my *Ultrafit* book, you're in luck! I tried not to repeat any of the same moves so you could have a bigger variety of exercises for your workouts with this book, *101 Ways to Work Out with Weights*.

My goal in writing *101 Ways to Work Out with Weights* is to provide you with 101 unique and effective resistance exercises using dumbbells, which can be executed whether you're new to exercise or at an advanced level. I've tried to make this process easy by composing complete workouts using these 101 exercises so you can see exactly how to put together a goal-oriented routine for yourself. I often claim to have what I call "EADD"—Exercise Attention Deficit Disorder. Sure, it's not real medical terminology; I just have trouble focusing on a workout when it's the same boring routine every single day. I'm easily distracted, and although I enjoy the results, it takes a truly interesting and inspirational routine to keep my attention. I'm not going to lie to you—weight lifting can be quite monotonous if you let it. So I'm constantly thinking of new exercises, trying crazy things, and mixing up my routines in order to look forward to going to my workouts. Some of the exercises that you'll see are actually variations on traditional movements, so many of the pictures and descriptions may seem vaguely familiar. I wanted to provide all fitness levels with a chance to use the exercises, so I provided both basic movements as well as exercises you may never have seen before. However, I'm hoping you'll really enjoy the combinations I've composed to create the most effective, exciting, and results-driven workouts possible. That is what makes working out fun!

✳ How I Got Started

My opinion on weight loss and body sculpting is that to build and create a body that is "lean and mean," you must be willing to put time and effort into the process. You must be patient. There is no magic pill you can take to look like the stars or fitness experts (they have *a lot* of behind-the-scenes help!). The only way to make changes in your metabolism and your body is through hard work and perseverance, and I definitely speak from experience. When I first moved to San Diego, I weighed 160 pounds, which is a lot for my frame and body type. I worked out all of the time, often teaching as many as three classes a day, and I maintained a full training schedule, which left me little time to focus on my own needs. As a result, I had terrible eating habits, and I got through each day depending on soda and sugar to give me enough energy. Finally, I had one of those "wake-up" moments and decided to make some serious changes. Within three months, due to a solid nutrition plan and an effective fitness regimen, I shed 40 pounds and sculpted a powerful 120-pound body bursting with energy and a balanced mental well-being.

After such a positive experience, I decided to start my own business, and Ultrafit Nutrition Systems was born. Sometimes the word *ultrafit* scares people; they think that it requires an extreme level of nutrition and fitness, which can be intimidating. But what being "ultrafit" really means is that a person has achieved his or her maximum potential, and this is different for everyone. We all need to set realistic goals so that when we make a commitment to ourselves, the probability of success serves to drive us forward. I want you to look at yourself in the mirror at the end of the day and love yourself, knowing that you're putting in 100 percent effort. Fitness and health are my passion, and I want to share them with you!

Good luck and God bless!

—Cindy Whitmarsh

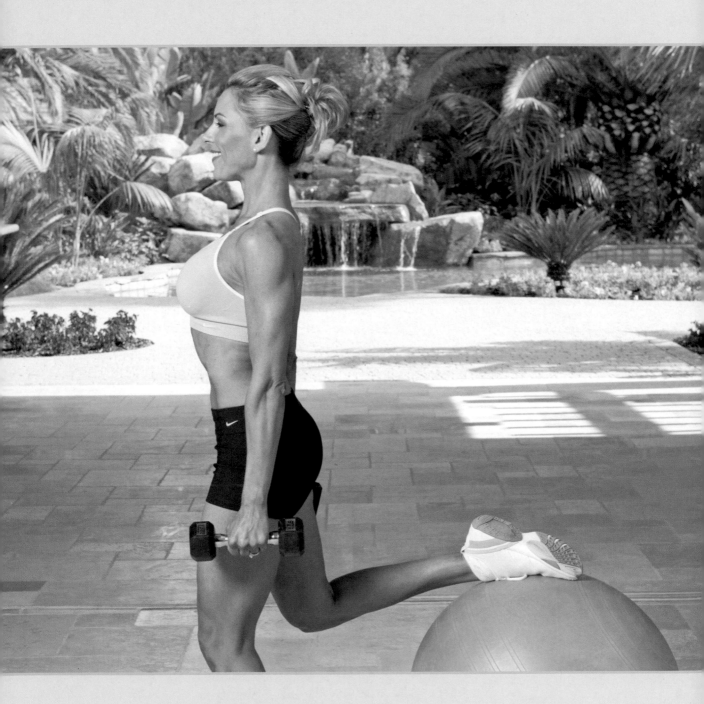

Why Weight Lifting Is Important for Women

Many women are afraid of weight lifting; they think they'll end up looking like the Incredible Hulk or, at the very least, too big or bulky. I can't even count the number of times a female client has said, "I don't lift weights because I don't want to bulk up." Oh my gosh! If I had a dollar for every time I've heard that phrase, I'd definitely be a rich woman!

It is very difficult for a woman to produce large muscles because women generally have high levels of the hormone estrogen. Estrogen is the hormone that produces female sex parts and our typically smaller amounts of lean tissue. Men typically produce more of the hormone testosterone, which produces the male sex parts and typically larger muscle tissue naturally. The improvements women experience will be made in muscle tone, strength, and endurance—not necessarily in size. As muscles become toned, the body begins to lose fat tissue and becomes firmer. When it comes to strength training, anything that is considered a healthy practice for men is also healthy for women. The fears about bulking up have created a cardio-only mind-set that serves only to burn calories, but rarely tones or tightens. Resistance exercises such as weight lifting increase your lean muscle mass, which in turn increases the amount of tissue in your body that naturally burns calories in a resting state (i.e., while you're sleeping!). If you do only cardio-based workouts, you'll burn calories and increase your cardiovascular output, but you risk the chance of burning muscle, thus slowing down your capability to burn calories and fat over the long run. This means you will risk the chance of slowing down your metabolism—*not* the effect you want. Cardio is only part of the job.

In addition, as women age, it becomes increasingly important that they focus on resistance exercises. Many changes in muscle tissue that are associated with age are caused by disuse. Just forcing your muscles to work on a regular basis can significantly improve their capacity to do work. You'll see improvements in circulation, coordination, balance, and bone and ligament strength. All of this is especially important for preventing loss of bone density and avoiding osteoporosis. You don't want to look like the Hunchback of Notre Dame, do you? Then get lifting! This book has an entire chapter dedicated to the topics of posture and core training, so make sure you don't skim through it! You can actually sabotage your own efforts because of your fears. Lift some weights, do cardio, and find the right nutrition. This combination will give you the strong, lean, healthy results you desire.

✳ Why Free Weights?

I like to use free weights when I lift for a couple of reasons:

1. **Cost:** Free weights aren't too expensive and are generally available at any sporting goods store. It's pretty easy to purchase a set to keep and use at home.

2. **Options:** There are a multitude of different exercises that you can do with free weights, such as the *101 Ways* described in this book. Also, you have the ability to easily work at different levels of intensity by using lighter or heavier weights.

3. **Challenge:** If you use proper form, free weights allow you a better range of motion than a machine does, which adds a new dimension of difficulty to your workouts and challenges multiple areas of the body at once. When you grow stronger, your body adapts to challenges at a quicker pace, and you're forced to challenge your muscles with different modalities and heavier weights to avoid a plateau. With free weights, the result is that more muscles are engaged and you get a more efficient workout. Although it may seem less efficient, you must go slowly, use good form, and use a controlled movement to work the muscles the right way to see your body change.

Expect results with consistent effort. In six weeks you could lose 4 to 6 percent body fat, and over twenty inches overall, if you are dedicated to doing at least thirty minutes of cardiovascular work four to six days a week, following a weight-lifting program two or three days a week, and sticking to a strict yet sensible nutrition plan. But I want you to keep in mind that sculpting your body, gaining muscle, and losing body fat requires consistency and determination to achieve optimal results. When you expect instant results (such as after just one week of hard work), you set yourself up for disappointment and potential failure. Let my advice, my careful planning, and my nutrition suggestions help guide you to the success you deserve. Check out the nutrition section and sample menu plan on pages 167 and 173 to help lead you on a healthy nutrition plan!

Set realistic goals. Follow the "S.M.A.R.T." concept and set goals that are Specific, Measurable, Achievable, Realistic, and Timely. If you've been a couch potato for the last year, don't jump right into an advanced program or you'll be in over your head. If you exercise regularly, don't start with a beginner program that provides little challenge or you'll quickly become bored. Setting realistic goals will help prevent the all-too-common tendency of starting something you either can't or don't want to finish.

Write it all down. What are your specific goals? How do you plan to achieve them? Why do you want to achieve them? Have you established a realistic time frame? Make sure you've thought through your plans and strategies, and aim to revisit your plans each day. Seeing your goals on paper will help keep you motivated and focused. In addition, keep a food and exercise log. The only person you're accountable to is yourself. If you're not seeing the results you want within a reasonable time frame, review your food and exercise log and try to determine what you might need to change. If you follow a program religiously, hitting a plateau may be a sign that you need to progress to the next level. The reason I keep bugging you about the whole package of good nutrition, cardio, and weight lifting is because I want you to see amazing results using the workouts I have provided you in this book!

Measure yourself to stay motivated and keep track of your results. Before you start a weight-lifting program, first take tape measurements and photos of yourself. You need to have a way to measure your progress, and the numbers on a scale are often misleading when you start to incorporate resistance training into your routine. The reason for this is that muscle weighs more than fat, and once on a new program, you may weigh more but go down a clothing size. I have my clients measure their biceps, forearm, shoulders, waist, hips, upper and lower thigh, and calf. Just make sure you are consistent with the sites you measure so you get a true reading each time!

If you have the ability to measure your body fat before starting a program, that is a great measurement of progress as well. I like my clients to find a piece of clothing that they want to fit into again, or to pin up an inspirational photo of themselves (or a figure they emulate). Keeping written records will help keep you motivated.

Avoid the overtraining syndrome. Always remember that sometimes less is more when it comes to working out. It's so incredibly important to have at least one rest day a week when your muscles and cardiovascular system have a chance to recover, repair, and rebuild. Overtraining can not only cause injuries and exhaustion, but it can also be the cause of either increased or decreased appetite, abnormal sleep patterns, and a compromised immune system. If you're wondering whether you're overtraining, turn to chapter 12, where I discuss what it means to have normal muscle soreness, and what it means if you have possibly worked out to the point of injuring yourself. And please, relaxing activities or hobbies such as hiking, biking, or yoga do not qualify as taking time off. Your day off is meant to be exercise-free!

Form, Technique, and Movement with Weights

The exercises in this book require the use of free weights. Free weights are relatively easy to use and will allow you to easily measure your progress as you modify the load (weight amount), volume (number of repetitions), and intensity of your program. Many of my female clients have expressed to me their fear of "looking stupid" in the gym, and they are often concerned that they won't be able to lift the weights correctly. Before you even get started with the workouts in this book, you need to take proper weight-training form and technique into account. I want you to learn the right way, and the wrong way, to lift weights. Using this mind-set, you'll be able to identify and correct errors and prevent future injuries.

Performing exercises correctly can help reduce the risk of common weight-training injuries such as sprains, strains, tendonitis, fractures, and dislocations. Continually using the same, improper weight-training technique can result in chronic injuries. Over time, you may find yourself with injuries involving the lower back, rotator cuff damage, muscle overload, bone stress injuries, or even nerve damage. If you don't use proper form when performing an exercise repetition, you might as well not perform the exercise at all because you are missing out on the intended rewards. Lifting lighter weight with good form will deliver more of the benefits of weight training than lifting heavier weights with bad form.

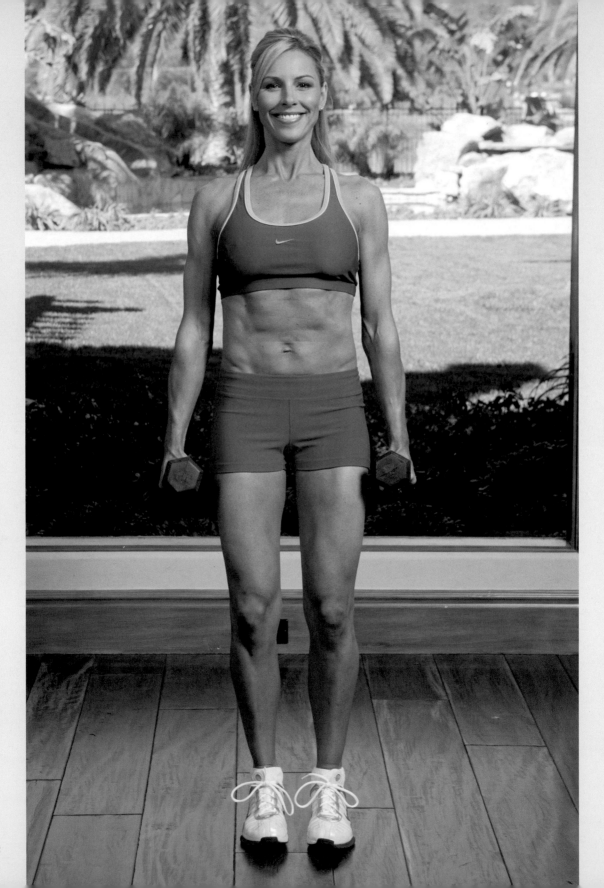

✳ Body Alignment

You must be conscious of your body alignment and posture when performing any exercise:

✔ When standing, feet should be shoulder-width apart with knees slightly bent. Picture a "midline" running from the top of your head down through the center of your body. As you exercise, keep your body weight balanced and evenly distributed in relation to your "midline."

✔ Proper posture has you standing tall with shoulders back and down (relaxed, not tense), your rib cage pulled in rather than extended, and your tummy pulled in tight.

✔ Your pelvis needs to be in a "neutral" alignment (your tailbone should be pointing down), and your abdominals should be contracted with the rib cage down. Remember, contracting your abdominal area (pulling the belly button in toward the spine) should not impede your ability to breathe in any way.

✔ Proper breathing techniques are essential when training. Never hold your breath. Exhale on the contraction and inhale during the release of each weight.

✳ Full Range of Motion

Precise weight-lifting form includes a full range of motion, which will lead to more uniform muscle development and increased flexibility:

✔ When performing exercises, the working muscles should extend throughout the full range of motion as dictated by muscle and joint flexibility.

✔ Be sure to maintain proper form and body alignment throughout the full range of motion.

✔ The speed at which you perform an exercise should be slow to moderate in order to allow you to maintain proper alignment and posture, while achieving a full range of motion. If you perform an exercise too quickly, the momentum of the movement won't allow you to maintain control, and injury can easily occur. As a suggestion, you can use a two- or four-count system with a pause at the top of the lift, and then a return to the starting position.

✓ It's important that you don't hyperextend your knee or elbow joints (don't "lock" them out) as this can increase potential injury to the joints.

✳ The Planes of Your Body

There are multiple planes (directions) in which your body can move. Throughout the book I will use the terms *saggital* and *frontal* planes. Visualize an invisible line drawn from the top and center of your head straight down between your eyes, nose, and directly through your belly button, cutting your body in half—that is the saggital plane. The frontal plane divides your body in half from the side, separating the front of your body from the back. It's a little weird to think of cutting your body in parts, but this is how we can describe which way your body should move or twist.

When a joint is stable in all planes, the muscles that surround it are balanced in their work efforts and function more efficiently. If a joint is not stable, then the muscles that are already strong in one plane work first and continue to grow stronger, while the weak muscles further deteriorate, which may cause ligaments to overstretch. This is why it is important to use proper body positioning and good posture when you are working out. It's also important to work your entire body to avoid muscular imbalances throughout your body!

✳ Muscular Isolation

When performing an exercise, you want to concentrate on isolating the targeted muscle or muscle group through both flexion and extension. In order to achieve proper isolation, you need to work the muscle or muscle group beyond fatigue so that the other supporting muscle groups compensate and take over.

It's important to feel the "negative" on every repetition. The negative movement is the eccentric movement (the releasing movement) of the exercise. For example, when performing a biceps curl, the pull or lifting of the weight toward your biceps is the concentric movement, and the lowering of the weight away from your biceps is the eccentric movement. The mistake many people make is to ignore the importance of the eccentric portion of the movement. Never let a weight simply drop quickly so you can bounce into the next rep. Let the contraction slowly and methodically open up as you return to the start position. This will allow you to train more efficiently, because you'll squeeze the full benefit out of every set.

✳ Resistance

You must use controlled and deliberate resistance in order to overload a muscle or muscle group and develop muscle strength. In order to see changes in muscular development, make sure you progressively increase the resistance used in your workouts. If you always lift the same weight, for the same number of repetitions and sets, you'll see initial changes, but never progress. Make sure that when the exercise you started with no longer fatigues the muscle or muscle group, you change the amount of weight you're using, the number of repetitions and sets, or both.

By remembering to maintain proper form and technique, you'll be able to correctly use the weight-training workouts outlined in this book. And when you perform the workouts regularly and combine them with a sensible nutrition plan, I guarantee you'll improve your strength, increase your muscle tone, lose fat, gain muscle mass, and improve your bone density.

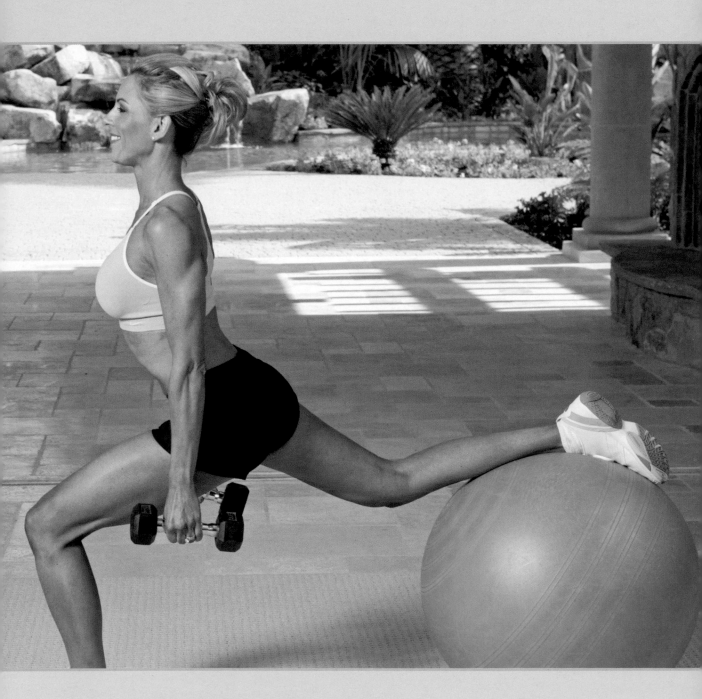

Determining Your Body Type

As you begin working out with weights, it's helpful to be able to recognize and work with your given genetic body type. A common mistake that many people make is to assume that all rules of dieting, exercise, and weight training apply to each and every individual in the same way. But the rules at hand will always vary, depending on your genetic makeup. When I moved to California from North Dakota forty pounds heavier than I am now, I was pear shaped, or an endomorph body type. I had a smaller waist and arms and larger glutes, hips, and outer thighs, and thicker legs. This is a hard body type to change because you have to reshape your body entirely. For me, it took concentrating on three different things. The first and most important was improving my nutrition to lose excess body fat. Second, I had to increase my upper-body size, strength, and shoulder width to make my hips and butt look smaller. Last, I had to decrease the size of my glutes and thighs to even out my pear-shaped body.

Regardless of age, race, or gender, you must set S.M.A.R.T. (Specific, Measurable, Achievable, Realistic, and Timely) fitness goals. Your genetics plays a huge role in your personal body type, so you should be aware of that when you are setting a fitness goal. If you have a smaller frame, trying to achieve a long body type resembling Julia Roberts might not be the best goal to set. Instead of setting goals based on someone you see on television or in a magazine, base your goals on developing a healthy body composition of reduced body fat and increased muscle mass, as well as an improved cardiovascular system and a healthy nutrition program.

Regardless, just getting moving and working out will be beneficial to both your mind and your body. Setting S.M.A.R.T. goals that work with your body type, not against it, will help you maintain a positive outlook. To this end, fitness trainers often use the generalized body-typing system that follows to assess individual needs and goals.

CHAPTER 3

✳ The Ectomorph

- Short upper body

- Long arms and legs

- Long, narrow feet and hands

- Very little fat storage and no difficulty losing body fat

- Narrow chest and round, narrow shoulders

- Indistinct buttocks

- Lean/lightly muscled

- Difficulty in gaining muscular definition and muscle mass without heavy weight training

Ectomorph Physique: An example of an ectomorph is Nicole Kidman. The ectomorph physique is usually pretty lean, and in some, it appears fragile and delicate. The bones are light, joints are small, and muscles are slight. The ectomorph is a linear physique—long limbs coupled with lack of muscle mass. The ectomorph is not naturally powerful and will have to work hard for every ounce of muscle and every bit of strength she or he can gain.

Ectomorph Training: The ectomorph's first objective is to gain muscle mass. Strength and endurance will need to be developed, and muscle mass develops very slowly. Stay with the basic exercises and include power moves that build maximum mass. Do an entire training workout, but take longer rest periods if you need to. Take in more calories than you are accustomed to, and use weight-gaining and protein drinks to supplement your food intake. Try not to expend too many calories by keeping cardio to a minimum; save them for muscle building. In chapter 13, I have designed a complete workout for the ectomorph body type. I suggest using heavier weights and fewer repetitions for this workout to help increase muscle mass faster. If you are a true ectomorph, you absolutely do not need to worry about bulking up! With your body type, it is almost impossible to put on enough muscle to have a bulky appearance. I chose exercises that will work the large muscle groups, like squats, leg extensions, hamstring curls, and full upper-body exercises. If you have time, I suggest performing three sets; the first set should be fifteen repetitions, the second set should be twelve reps, and the third set should be ten reps. You'll get the best results from this system if you pyramid your sets, which means increasing the weight for each set.

✳ The Endomorph

- Round, softer shape

- Short, heavy legs

- Round face

- Short neck

- Narrow shoulders and a large chest

- Wide hips

- Underdeveloped muscles

- Weight loss is difficult

- Gains muscle easily

- Heavy fat storage, usually concentrated in the lower body (hips and abdomen)

Endomorph Physique: An example of an endomorph is Jennifer Lopez. The endomorph's physique is often round and soft (the "apple" shape). Often, much of the mass is concentrated in the abdominal area. Many endomorphs desire a leaner, more defined look, and they should be taking in six to seven smaller meals throughout the day to help boost the metabolism and burn fat and calories. Cardiovascular work is essential for endomorphs looking to trim down. Meanwhile, weight training should contain sets of several repetitions at a moderate weight, with limited time spent between sets.

Endomorph Training: The endomorph should be concerned with decreasing body fat while maintaining lean muscle mass. In chapter 13, I have designed a workout for the endomorph body type. I suggest training with heavier weights for the upper body, and doing high repetitions with lighter weights for the lower body. This will help the endomorph increase upper-body size and balance out the total body. I also suggest having a relatively short rest period in between sets in order to keep the heart rate up in the "fat-burning zone" and maximize caloric expenditure. This should all be in addition to a controlled reduced-calorie diet that contains the necessary nutritional balance of protein, carbohydrates, and fats.

✳ The Mesomorph

- Athletic, muscular body

- Large chest (larger than waist)

- Long torso

- Broad shoulders

- Excellent posture

- No difficulty losing body fat or sculpting for definition (gains muscle easily)

- Very strong

Mesomorph Physique: An example of a mesomorph is Demi Moore. The mesomorph physique is the typical "hourglass." Mesomorphs have the tendency to be muscular and developed, maintaining the best attributes of both the ectomorphs and the endomorphs. Mesomorphs must basically follow the general guidelines of healthy eating and exercise to maintain their physiques.

Mesomorph Training: The mesomorph needs to include a variety of exercises in her program so that her muscles develop proportionately and are shapely rather than bulky. A combination of heavy power moves and a variety of shaping exercises will provide for a better quality, proportion, and symmetry of the physique. The mesomorph responds well to training, so superlong sessions are not needed. The workout that I planned in chapter 13 for the mesomorph body type consists of more cardio-like exercises and exercises using your own body weight. The cardio will help to burn extra calories, and because mesomorphs build muscle quickly, using their own body weight is a sufficient way to train.

Most individuals tend to have characteristics from a combination of two categories (such as endo-meso or meso-ecto). For example, I am now a mix of ectomorph and mesomorph. I have long muscles, but after my weight loss, I'm now in better proportion than with my previous endomorph body. The main focus here should be looking at your parents and then looking at yourself openly and honestly in the mirror. Your "ideal" body type may not be a realistic expectation. Accepting the beautiful and positive aspects of your body is your first step toward achieving your ultimate fitness goals.

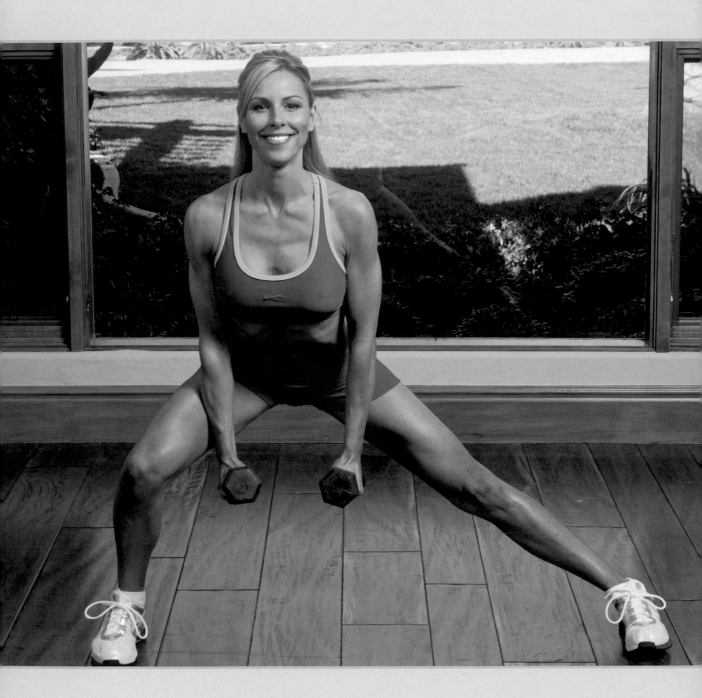

The Warm-Up and Its Importance (Exercises 1–6)

CHAPTER 4

My Ultrafit Program has locations all over Southern California, so I spend a majority of my time in and around gyms. I watch members walk right into the weight room or jump into a class straight from the street. They're so eager to get started, and so impatient, that they neglect to go through a proper warm-up (and then they wonder how they get injured!). Some of the professional athletes I work with do the same thing, and they've had the information drilled into their heads time and time again by their own coaches! And I'm not talking about stretching—the jury is still out on whether stretching prior to a workout is harmful or beneficial. The warm-up needs to not only be active, but functional. Your goal is to perform movements similar to what you'll be doing during your workout, but with no resistance and very low intensity. You want to increase the blood flow to your muscles, so that you can help prevent any injury, and so your body is prepared to perform at peak levels.

I suggest two stages of warm-up:

1. Perform at least five minutes of cardiovascular activity (such as cycling, walking, using the elliptical machine, stair climbing, etc.). I want you to raise your body's core temperature and get blood pumping into your muscle fibers at a higher volume. You need to enhance the elasticity of your muscles before you do any lifting routine. Some people need more of a warm-up than others. Get to know your body and the amount of time it needs to feel warm and loose.

2. Use light weights (one to five pounds) to perform functional movements that are muscle-specific and mimic the exercises you have planned for your workout.

I have designed six warm-up exercises using light weights that mimic all of the 101 exercises in this book in some shape or form. The warm-up exercises should be performed slowly and with light weights to ensure proper form and to prevent injury. I suggest using one- to five-pound dumbbells, depending on your fitness level. It's ideal to do some type of cardiovascular warm-up first to increase your body's core temperature.

1 Torso Twist (All Levels)

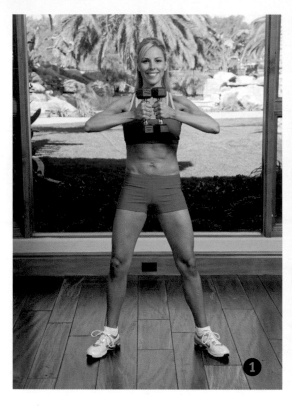

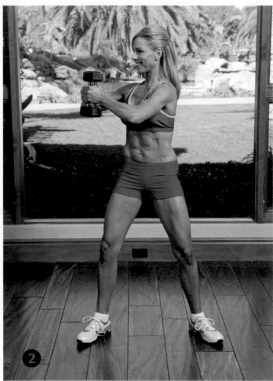

Benefits: Warms up body's core (center of body)
---

① Stand tall with a slight bend in your knees, holding dumbbells in both hands directly in front of your chest, keeping your elbows bent. This is your starting position.

② Begin by pulling in your abs and slowly rotate your torso and the dumbbells from side to side continually.

③ Repeat movement for 30 repetitions, with one side to the other equaling 1 rep.

Alternating Front Punch (All Levels)

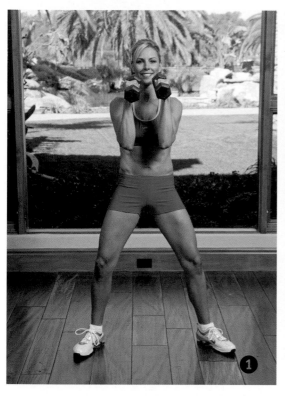

◎

Benefits: Warms up upper body

---

① Start by standing with your legs slightly wider than hip-width apart, with knees and toes turned out and your knees slightly bent. Hold dumbbells in your hands directly in front of your shoulders with your elbows bent and forearms in vertical position. This is your starting position.

② While keeping your heels on the ground, and alternating arms, punch your arms diagonally in front, keeping your arms parallel to the ground and a slight bend in your elbows as you extend.

③ Repeat the alternating cross punch for 30 repetitions, with one side to the other equaling 1 rep.

3 Wood Chop (All Levels)

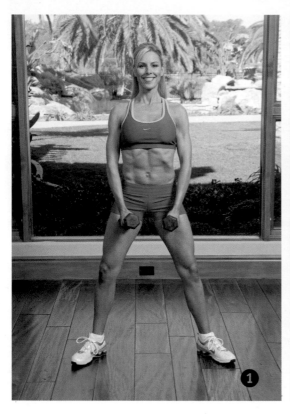
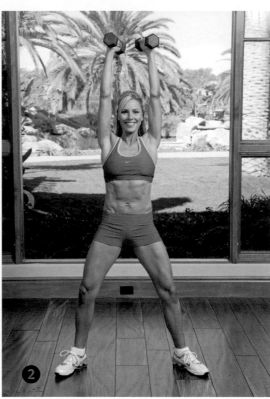

① Start by standing with your legs slightly wider than hip-width apart, with knees and toes turned out and your knees slightly bent. Hold dumbbells in your hands with your arms extended toward the floor. This is your starting position.

② Initiate movement by pulling in your abs and lifting the dumbbells over your head with straight arms while slightly leaning backward to stretch your core.

Benefits: Warms up entire body and stretches core

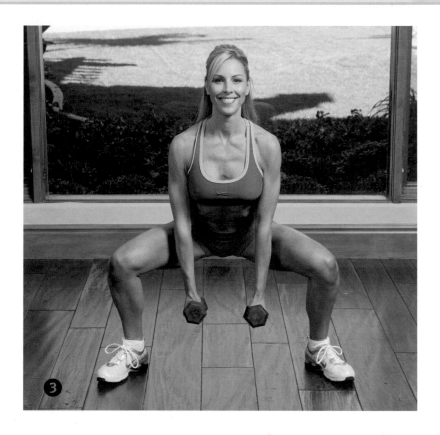

③ Next bring the dumbbells toward the floor while bending your knees into a squat position with your thighs parallel to the ground and knees at a 90-degree angle but no lower. Keep your spine in a neutral position, as straight as you can. Do not drop your head.

④ Repeat the wood chopping movement for 30 repetitions, 15 up and 15 down.

4

Squat into Overhead Shoulder Press (All Levels)

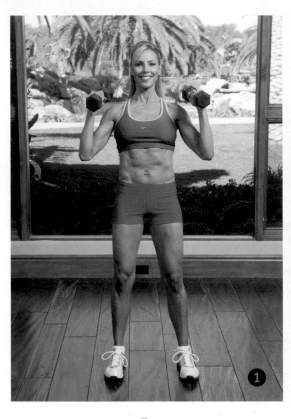

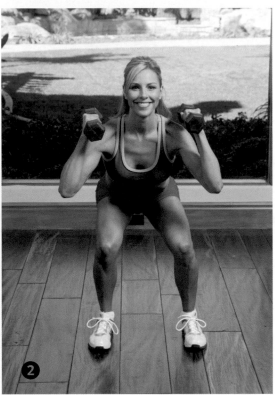

Benefits: Warms up entire body and stretches core

(1) Hold dumbbells in your hands slightly to the sides of your shoulders, with your elbows bent and forearms in vertical position. This is your starting position.

(2) Keeping your spine neutral and abs tight, squat down, keeping the dumbbells by your shoulders, until your thighs are parallel to the ground and your knees are at a 90-degree angle but no lower.

4

③ Stand up slowly by pushing off with your heels. As you are standing, go directly into a shoulder press, pressing the dumbbells overhead.

④ Return to the starting position and repeat for 30 repetitions.

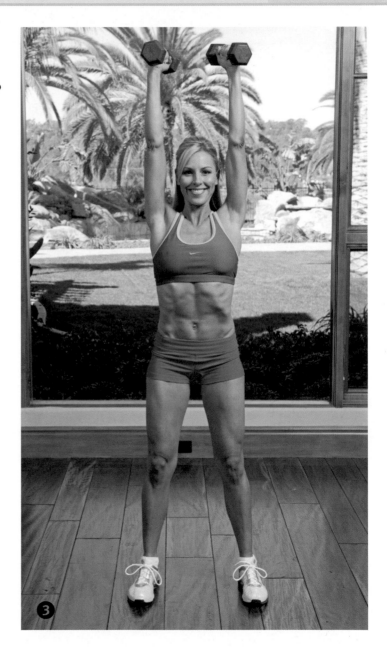

5 Alternating Front Lunge and Torso Twist (Intermediate)

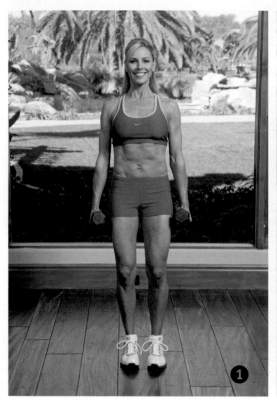

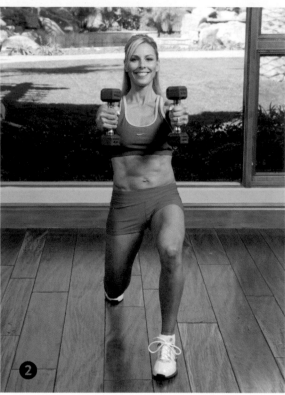

Benefits: Warms up the lower body
and stretches and tones core muscles

(1) Begin by standing with dumbbells in
your hands and your arms extended
down by your sides. This is your starting position.

(2) Extend your arms in front of you so they
are parallel to the ground and simultane-
ously perform a front lunge by stepping
your left leg out, bending your knee to a
90-degree angle, and placing your weight
on the heel of your left foot.

5

③ Hold this front lunge position and perform a torso rotation by rotating your torso, along with the dumbbells, to the same side as the leg that is forward in the lunge. Then bring your torso and dumbbells back to the center lunge position.

④ To finish this exercise, stand back up by pushing off the heel of the front foot that is in the lunge and bring your arms and dumbbells back to your sides in the standing position. Repeat the movement on the right side and then alternate sides so you complete 15 repetitions on each leg.

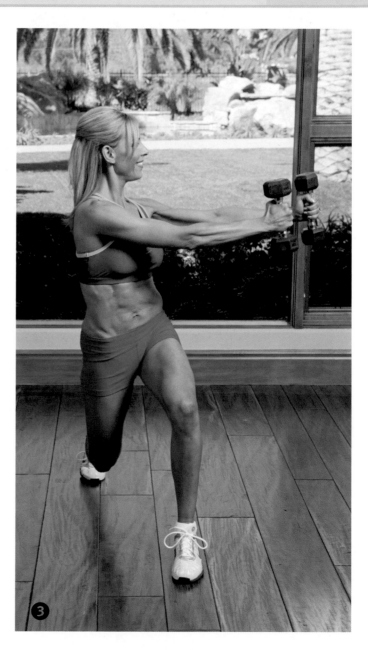

Alternating Side Lunge and Shoulder Press (Intermediate)

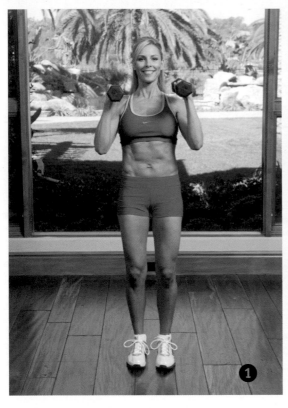

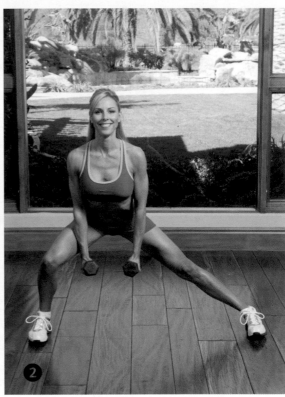

◎

Benefits: Warms up entire body

---

① Stand and hold dumbbells in your hands directly in front of your shoulders with your elbows bent and forearms in vertical position. This is your starting position.

② Keeping your spine neutral and abs tight, perform a side lunge with the right leg stepping out sideways and bending so your knee and toes stay straight forward, and your knee is directly over your heel. Your lunge should end with your thigh parallel to the ground. Your left leg should remain straight, and your arms and dumbbells should reach for your right foot.

③ Stand back up by pushing off your heel towards your starting position and begin an overhead shoulder press with both arms.

④ Return to your starting position and switch sides, alternating until you have performed 10 repetitions on each leg.

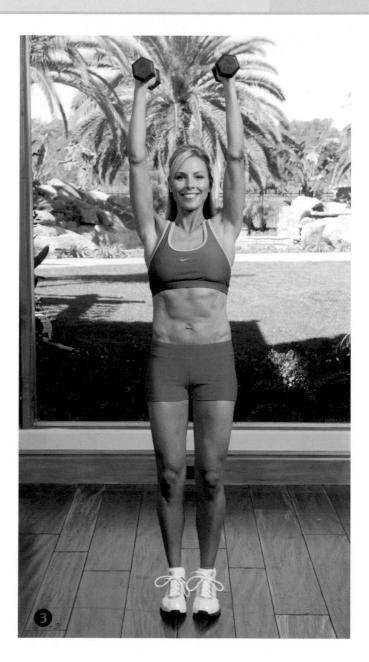

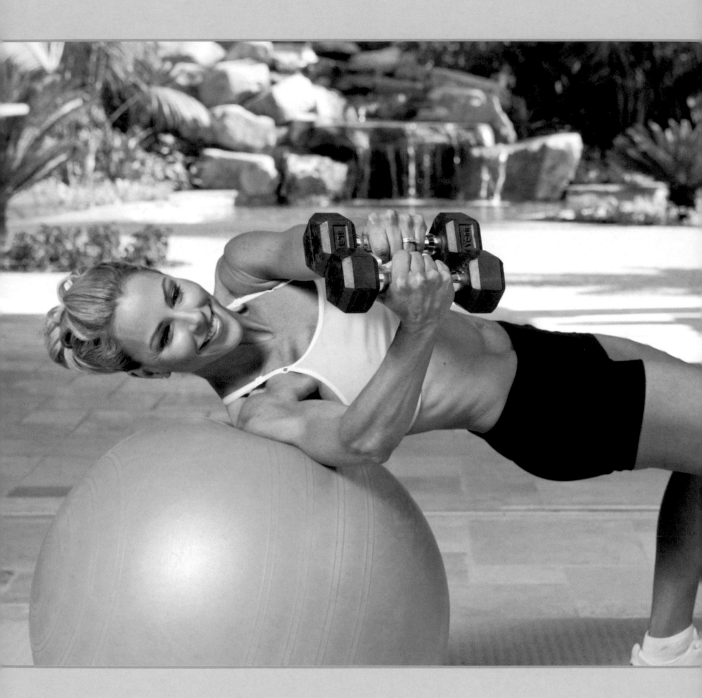

Weights for the Upper Body (Exercises 7–26)

I've designed this chapter as a guide to specifically show a variety of ways that you can work out your upper body with weights. Lifting weights to work out your upper body will improve your posture, help you become stronger in your functional everyday activities (so you don't hurt yourself doing the most mundane chore!), and help give your body a leaner and more balanced physique.

I've included a variety of exercises using beginner, intermediate, and advanced moves. Any of the exercises that use a flat bench may be performed using a stability ball instead of a bench. This will add an element of core challenge to the exercise (thus increasing the difficulty of the movement). (Check out chapter 7 for more exercises using the stability ball.) I have given you a suggested amount of repetitions for each of these exercises. The beginning of your routine will involve some trial and error since you first have to determine the correct amount of weight to start with. To make this determination, perform repetitions with gradually increasing weights. As you come to your last three repetitions with a specific weight, your muscles should be fatigued—this is the weight with which you should start. If I recommend twelve to fifteen reps and you can easily go for twenty, you should increase the amount of weight you are using at the start. In chapter 13, I've designed specific workouts using all 101 exercises so that you can see how to use the exercises in a complete workout.

And most important, don't forget to warm up! I've provided you with some examples of warm-up exercises in chapter 4. Have fun!

CHAPTER 5

7

BACK
Incline Bench Row (Beginner)

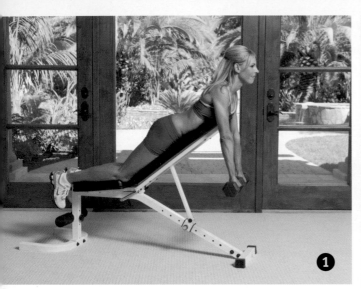

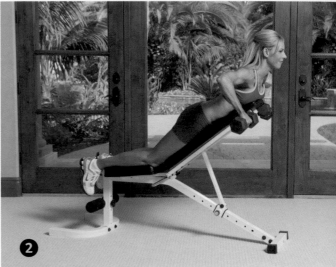

①

②

◎

Benefit: Strengthens upper back

① Bring your bench to a seated incline position. While holding your dumbbells in your hands, kneel down facing the back of the bench so your chest and thighs press against the incline. Your arms should extend toward the floor. This is your starting position.

② Begin the exercise by keeping your neck neutral and contracting your shoulder blades as if you are pinching a pencil between them. Next, pull the dumbbells up, leading with your elbows and stopping when your back is contracted.

③ Return to the starting position and repeat for 12 to 15 repetitions.

Dumbbell Pullover (Beginner)

8

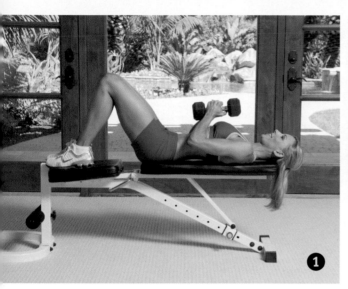

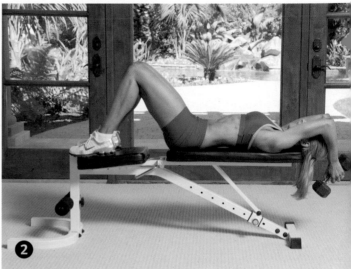

Benefit: Strengthens upper back
---

(1) Start with one heavier dumbbell in your hands and keep it close to your chest as you lie down on a flat bench. Bring your feet up on the bench. This is your starting position.

(2) Begin the exercise by lifting and reaching your dumbbell back over your head and down until you feel your back contracting. Squeeze your shoulder blades together, contracting your back while also keeping a natural curve in your back.

(3) Return to the starting position and repeat for 12 to 15 repetitions.

9

One-Arm Row from Plank Position (Advanced)

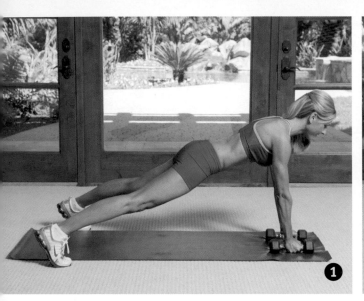

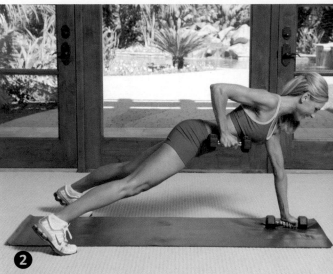

◎

Benefits: Strengthens back and core

(1) Hold dumbbells in your hands and come down onto your hands and knees, with your knees slightly wider than hip-width apart. Straighten your arms so your dumbbells are on the ground directly over your shoulders. While contracting your abs, lift your knees up so your body is elevated and horizontal to the ground with your toes anchoring. This is your starting position.

(2) From this prone plank position, perform a one-arm dumbbell row by pulling your right dumbbell up, leading with your elbow, and squeeze your latissimus dorsi (side of back).

(3) Return to the starting position and repeat on the same side until you complete 12 to 15 repetitions. Then complete 12 to 15 reps on the opposite side.

Straight-Arm Pullover with One Leg Out (Advanced)

10

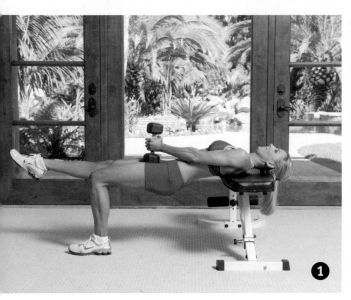 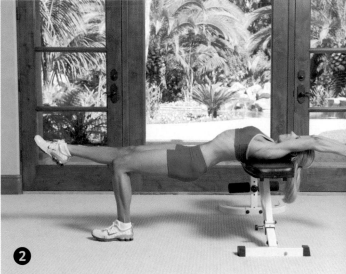

◎

Benefits: Strengthens back and core

① Get into position by holding one dumbbell in your hands, close to your chest, and bend down to the side of a flat bench. Lean back so your head and neck are supported by the flat bench, with your hips up in the air squeezing your glutes. Keep your abs tight. From this position, extend your right leg out so it is parallel to the ground. Extend your arms towards your thighs and stop when your arms are extended, holding your dumbbell by your thighs. This is your starting position.

② Begin the exercise by lifting the dumbbell with straight arms back behind your head and toward the floor while squeezing your shoulder blades together and contracting your back.

③ Return to the starting position. Repeat half of your repetitions with your right leg out and then switch legs and do the other half with your left leg out. Complete a total of 12 to 16 reps.

11

CHEST
Dumbbell Push-Up (Beginner)

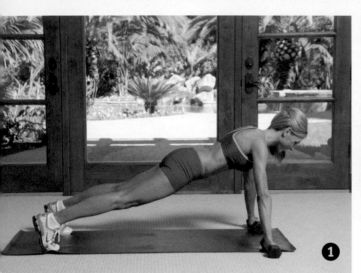

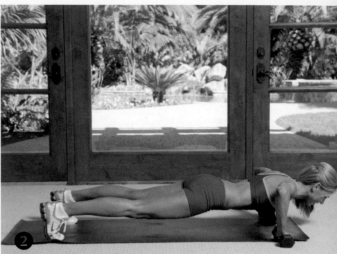

◎

Benefits: Strengthens chest and upper body

---

① Begin this exercise holding two dumb-bells in your hands (preferably using dumbbells with square edges for more support). You may do the push-up from your knees, making it more of a beginner exercise, or from your toes. Holding your dumbbells in your hands, bring your body down into a prone position with your weights under your shoulders and either your knees or toes touching the ground. This is your starting position.

② Perform the push-up by first tightening your abs and lowering your body toward the ground, using the dumbbells for wrist support.

③ Squeeze your chest and push yourself back to your starting position. Repeat this exercise for 12 to 15 repetitions.

Multi-Repetition Incline Chest Press (Beginner)

◎

Benefits: Strengthens chest and shoulders

① Sit on a seated incline bench with your feet firmly planted on the foot rest, holding dumbbells to each side of your chest with bent elbows. This is your starting position.

② Keep your back against the incline bench to keep a neutral spine and try not to arch as you lift. Press the right dumbbell up, squeezing your chest, and then lower it. Next, press the left dumbbell up and down.

③ Finish the first set by performing two double-arm presses up and down twice. One set will equal single, single, double, double.

④ Repeat this series of repetitions for a total of 12 to 15 reps.

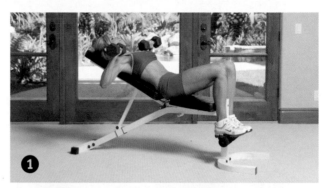

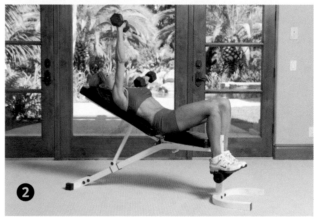

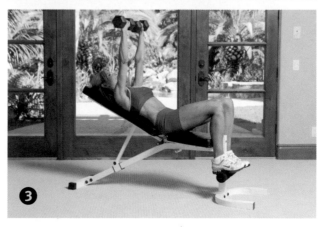

13 Roll-Out Push-Up (Advanced)

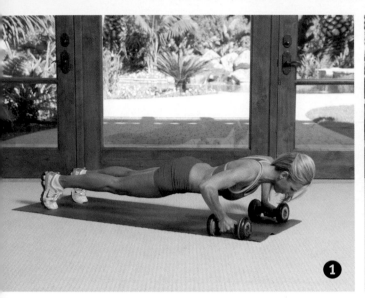 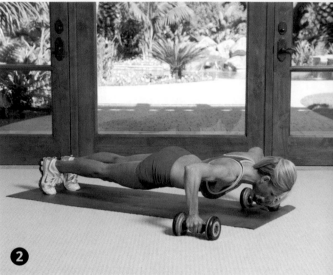

─────── ◎ ───────

Benefits: Strengthens chest, upper body, and core

(1) Begin this exercise holding two dumbbells in your hands (preferably using dumbbells with round edges for more support). You may do the push-up from your knees, making it more of an intermediate exercise, or from your toes. Holding your dumbbells in your hands, bring your body down into a downward-facing position with your weights under your shoulders, and either your knees or toes touching the ground. This is your starting position.

(2) Begin this exercise by pulling in your abs and keeping a neutral spine, then laterally roll one dumbbell out until your arm is extended almost straight out and stop. Drop your chest toward the ground, performing a pushup, tighten your chest and core, come back up, and roll the dumbbell back to the center and starting position.

(3) Repeat this exercise on the other side and continue alternating each arm out and push-ups until you have completed 10 on each side.

Dumbbell Fly with Supinated Wrists (Advanced)

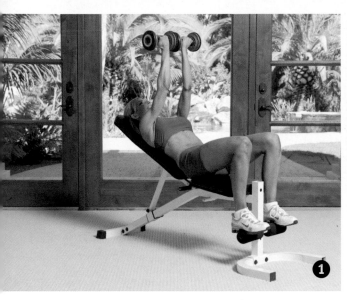

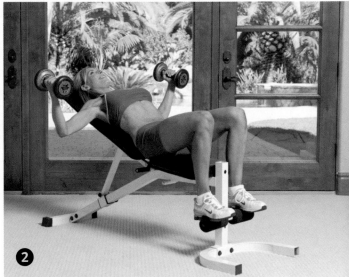

1 **2**

Benefits: By turning your wrists, you give your chest a better contraction and a different feel than when you just go up and down with your palms facing each other throughout the movement.

(1) Hold dumbbells in your hands and lie face-up on either a flat bench or a seated incline bench with your feet flat on the floor or on the foot rest. Fully extend your arms above your chest, palms facing your head. Keep a slight bend in your elbows. This is your starting position.

(2) Slowly lower the dumbbells to the outside of your chest, turning your wrists outward as you go, until your hands are about even with your chest. Bring the dumbbells back up, keeping your pinkies up, and touch the dumbbells together at the top of the movement. Squeeze your chest, then slowly lower and repeat.

(3) Repeat the exercise for 12 to 15 repetitions.

15

SHOULDERS

Dumbbell Upright Row into Alternating Single-Arm Press (Beginner)

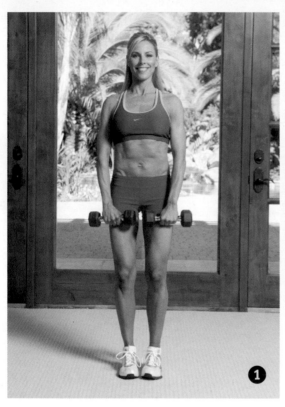

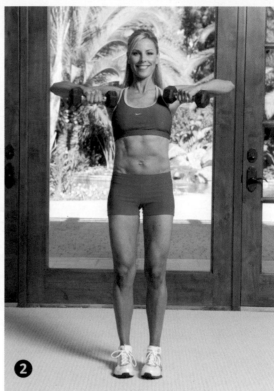

◎

Benefit: Strengthens shoulders

(1) Hold dumbbells in your hands with your arms down in front of your thighs and your palms facing your legs. This is your starting position.

(2) Initiate the movement by bending your elbows and lifting from your elbows with the dumbbells following until your elbows are at the top of the movement and the dumbbells are lower.

15

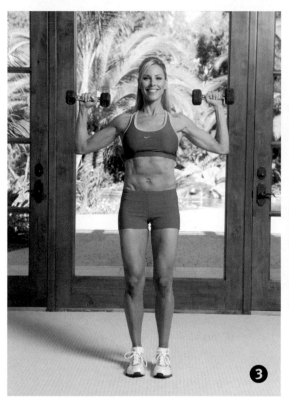 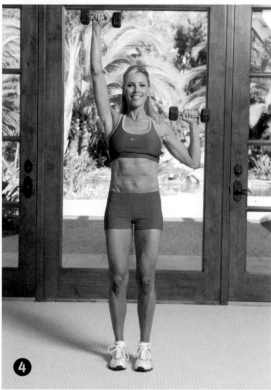

(3) Contract your shoulder blades behind and lift the dumbbells up so they are at the sides of your shoulders.

(4) This is the third part of the exercise. Perform a single-arm shoulder press by pushing one dumbbell straight up, contracting your shoulder, bringing it back down, and then switching sides.

(5) Return both dumbbells to the starting position and repeat. One repetition is one upright row, both single-arm overhead presses, and then back down. Repeat this complete exercise for 12 to 15 repetitions.

16 Shoulder 3-Phase Move (Beginner)

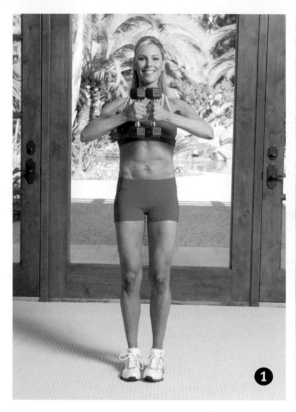
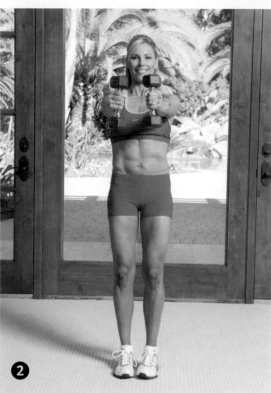

❶   ❷

Benefit: Strengthens shoulders

1. Hold lighter dumbbells directly in front of your chest with your elbows bent and your forearms parallel to the floor. This is your starting position.

2. Begin the movement by extending your elbows until your arms are straight out in front of you.

3. Then bring the weights out to your sides, keeping your arms straight and parallel to the floor in a crosslike pattern.

④ From this point, perform the exercise in the reverse pattern. Repeat this exercise for 12 to 15 repetitions.

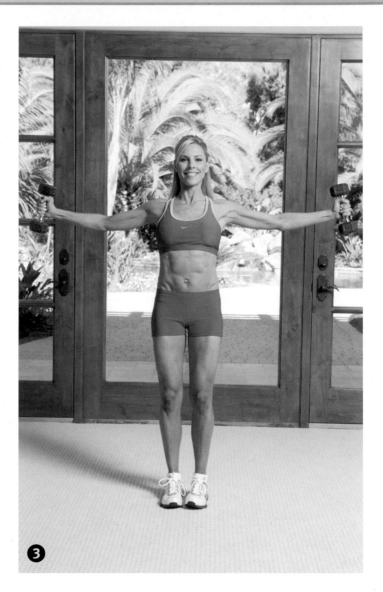

17 Balancing Single-Leg Rear Delt Fly (Intermediate/Advanced)

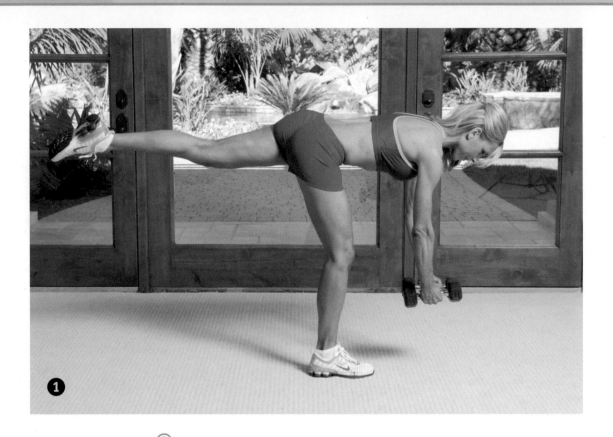

①

Benefits: Strengthens rear deltoids, core, and legs; improves balance and posture

① Stand and hold dumbbells in your hands at your sides. Next, contract your abs and slowly lift your left leg up and back while bending forward at the same time until your chest and back leg are parallel to the ground. (It is okay if your back leg is a bit lower for flexibility reasons.) The dumbbells and your arms will hang vertically. This is your starting position.

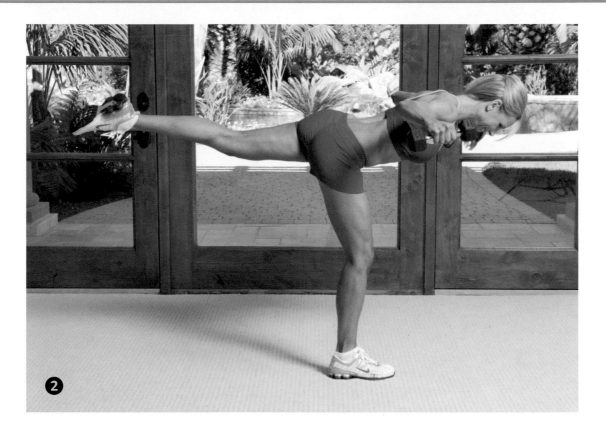

(2) While contracting your abs and keeping your leg raised behind you, lift the dumbbells while laterally contracting your rear deltoids. Lead with your elbows slightly bent until your arms are parallel to the ground. Return the dumbbells back down to your starting position.

(3) Repeat this exercise with your left leg raised for half of your reps, and then switch legs for the second half of your repetitions. Complete 12 to 16 repetitions total.

Note: To make this exercise more intermediate, you may keep your feet together on the floor instead of raised and balanced behind you.

18 Side-Lying, Internal-Rotation Rear Deltoid Raise (Intermediate/Advanced)

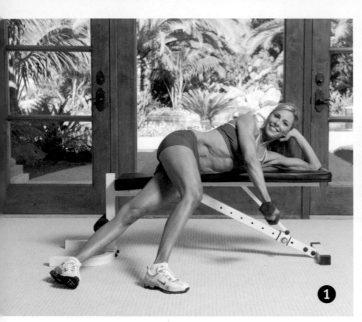
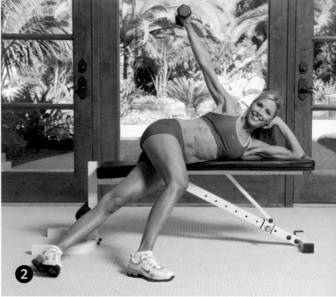

◎

Benefits: Strengthens the rear deltoid
and medial deltoid

---

① Start by lying on your side on a flat bench. Hold a dumbbell in the hand of your working arm (allow your nonworking arm to rest comfortably along the bench), and then extend your arm in front of you, pointing your pinky finger up and your arm slightly toward the floor. For balance, split your legs touching the floor—bottom leg in back and top leg in front. This is your starting position.

② With your arm slightly bent, raise the dumbbell toward the ceiling. When your arm reaches roughly 30 degrees below perpendicular to the floor, stop and hold. Squeeze the contraction for 1 to 2 seconds. Slowly lower the dumbbell back to the starting position.

③ Repeat this exercise for 12 to 15 repetitions on each side.

◎

Note: Use a light dumbbell for this motion to avoid injury. Use slow movements (do not jerk your arm) to isolate your shoulder—not your back. Keep your hand and wrist stable; don't turn the dumbbell.

BICEPS

Seated Single-Arm Concentration Curl (Beginner)

19

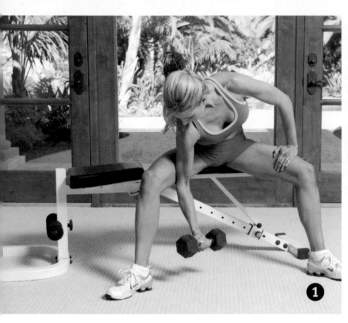 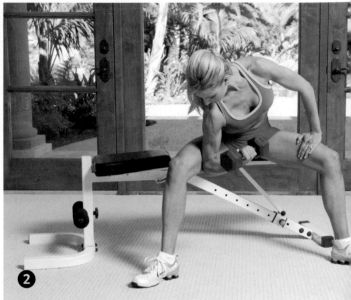

① ②

◎

Benefit: Strengthens biceps

---

① Sit on a bench, and hold one heavier dumbbell in your right hand. Plant your feet on the floor and place your legs out wide, turning your knees and feet out. Bend over, holding the dumbbell, and dig your right elbow into the side of your right thigh with your arm extended down toward the ground. This is your starting position.

② First contract your biceps and bend your elbow, bringing the dumbbell toward your shoulder. Squeeze your biceps at the top of the contraction. Pause for 2 seconds and return.

③ Repeat the exercise for 12 to 15 repetitions on each arm.

20 Seated Incline Crunch and Biceps Curl (Beginner)

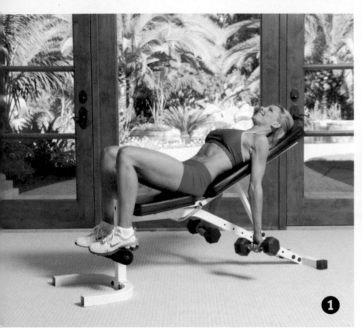
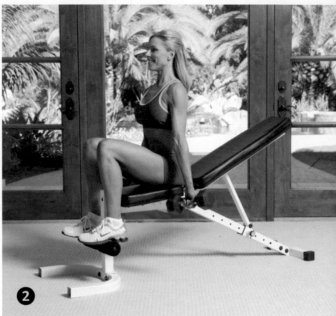

❶ ❷

◎

Benefits: Strengthens biceps and abs

---

① Lie on an incline bench and hold a medium to heavy dumbbell in each hand, with your arms resting down by your sides. This is your starting position.

② Perform an abdominal crunch by lifting your torso off the bench and crunching your abs.

③ Once you are up, perform biceps curls with both arms by pulling the dumbbells towards your shoulders; squeeze your biceps at the top. Hold for 2 seconds, and then extend your arms back down to your sides, and lie back down on the incline bench.

④ Repeat the exercise for 12 to 15 repetitions.

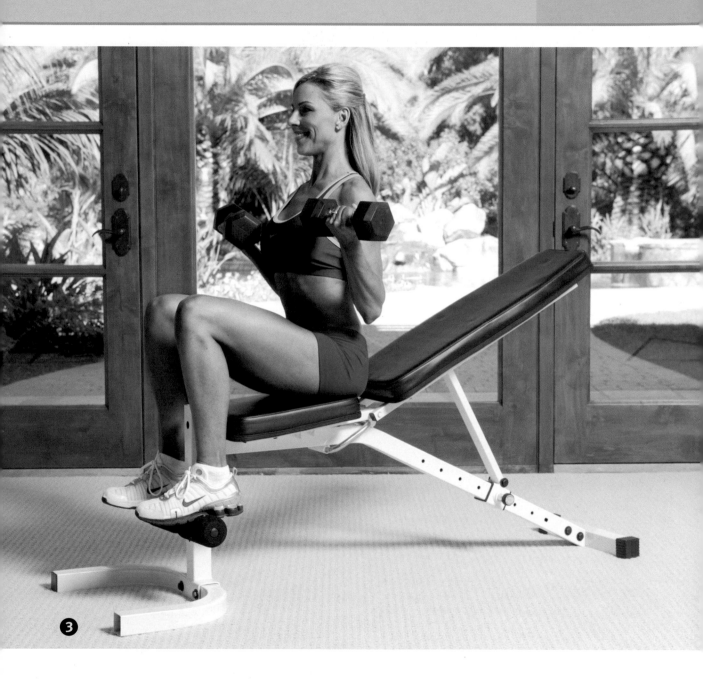

❸

21 Side-Lunge Single-Arm Concentration Curl (Advanced)

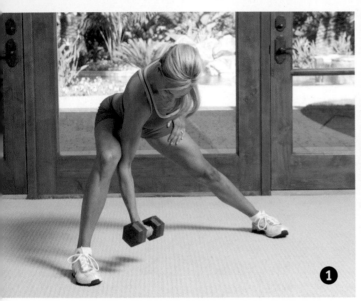

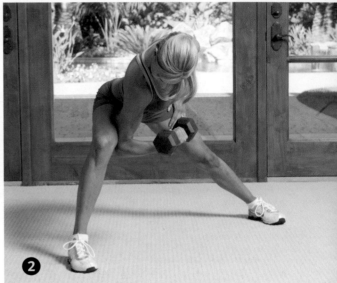

1

2

◎

Benefits: Strengthens legs, glutes, core, and biceps

① Start by holding one medium to heavy dumbbell in your right hand. Begin by stepping your right leg out to the side in a bent-knee lunge, keeping your knees and toes facing forward and your knee directly over your heel. Your left leg should be straight. Bend over and place your right elbow into the side of your right thigh and extend your arm down,

holding your dumbbell. Keep your left hand on your left leg for balance. This is your starting position.

② First contract your biceps and bend your elbow, bringing the dumbbell towards your shoulder. Squeeze your biceps at the top of the contraction. Pause for 2 seconds and return. Stay in the side lunge position for all of the repetitions on this side.

③ Complete 12 to 15 repetitions on your right side, and then switch lunges and arms to work your left side.

Balancing Single-Leg Alternating Biceps Curl (Advanced)

22

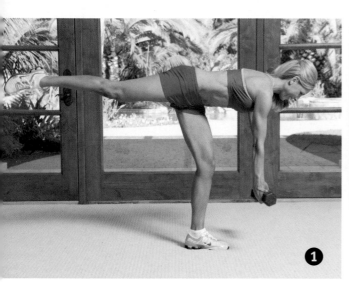 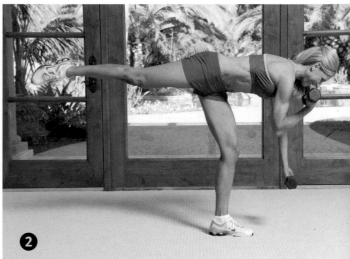

◎

Benefits: Strengthens biceps, core,
and legs, and improves balance

---

1. Stand with your hands at your sides, holding medium-weight dumbbells. Next, contract your abs and slowly lift your right leg up and back while bending forward at the same time, until your chest and back leg are parallel to the ground. (It is okay if your back leg is a bit lower for flexibility reasons.) Let your arms hang down at your sides, holding the dumbbells. This is your starting position.

2. While maintaining a tight core position and balancing, complete alternating biceps curls by bending your right arm first, lifting your dumbbell to your shoulder, squeezing your biceps, and then coming back down.

3. Continue by alternating right- and left-side biceps curls until you have completed half of your repetitions with the right leg raised. Switch to your left leg raised and finish the rest of your reps. Repeat this exercise for 12 to 16 total repetitions.

23

TRICEPS
Skull Crushers (Beginner)

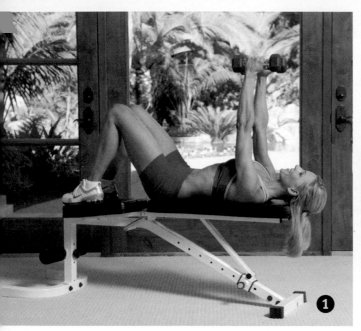

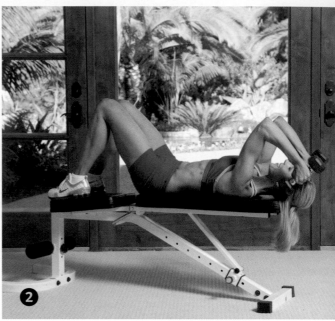

Benefit: Strengthens triceps
---

(1) Lie on a bench holding dumbbells in your hands with your arms extended above your chest.

(2) Exhale, bend your elbows, and slowly lower the dumbbells toward the back of your head. Keep your elbows in; only your forearms are moving down and up. Push them halfway back up and then bring them back down. Finish by returning the dumbbells to an extended position. Contract your abs and make sure you do not use momentum to move the dumbbells.

(3) Repeat the skull crushers for 12 to 15 repetitions.

Bent-Over Double-Arm Triceps Kickback (Beginner)

24

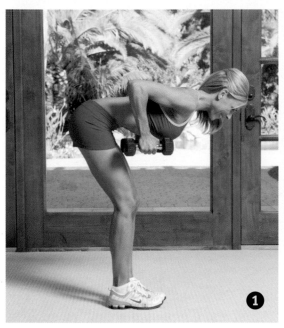

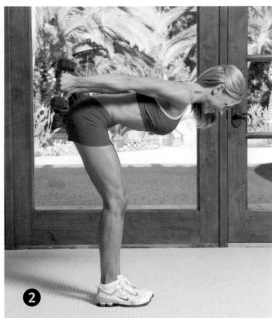

1

2

◎

Benefits: Strengthens triceps and core

---

① Stand with dumbbells in your hands, contract your abs, and bend over from your hips until your chest is parallel to the ground. Pull your elbows up so they are directly next to your sides, with the dumbbells in your hands hanging toward the ground. This is your starting position.

② Initiate the movement by extending your elbows and forearms toward your back and squeezing your triceps.

③ Bring the dumbbells back to the starting position and repeat for 12 to 15 repetitions.

25 Supine Bridge Single-Leg Triceps Extension (Advanced)

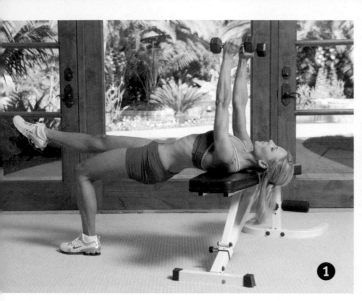 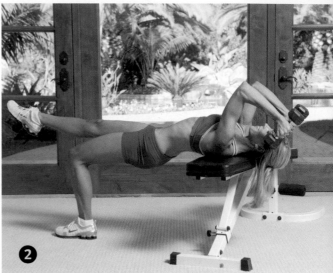

① **②**

◎

Benefits: Strengthens triceps, core,
and quadriceps and improves balance

① Sit on the side of a bench, holding dumbbells in your hands and resting them on your thighs. Start by sliding down toward the ground until your head and neck are supported by the bench. Walk your feet out so your heels are planted, your hips are raised, and your glutes are tight. From this position, extend your arms straight up toward the ceiling and then extend one leg out straight, while keeping your hips raised and your glutes and abs tight. This is your starting position.

② While maintaining a stable position, perform the triceps extension. Exhale, bend your elbows, and slowly lower the dumbbells towards the back of your head, keeping your elbows in; only your forearms are moving down and up. Push them halfway back up and then bring them back down. Finish by returning the dumbbells to an extended position. Contract your abs and make sure you do not use momentum to move the dumbbells.

③ Complete 12 to 16 reps total. Do half of your repetitions with one leg up and then switch the raised leg for the second half of the repetitions.

Balancing Single-Leg Triceps Kickback (Intermediate/Advanced)

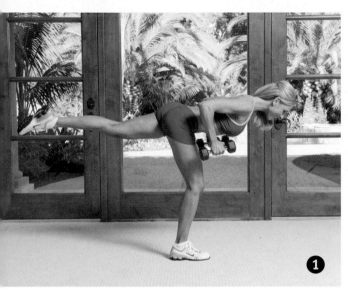
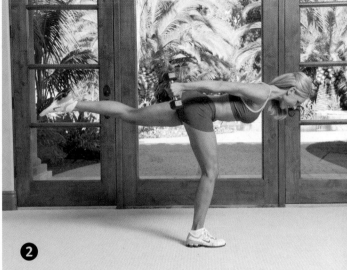

① **②**

Benefits: Strengthens triceps, core, and legs; improves balance and posture

① Stand with your hands at your sides, holding dumbbells. Next, contract your abs and slowly lift your left leg up and back while bending forward at the same time until your chest and back leg are parallel to the ground. (It is okay if your back leg is a bit lower for flexibility reasons.) Bring your elbows back and up so they are directly next to your sides and the dumbbells are hanging down. This is your starting position.

② While maintaining a tight core position and balancing, extend your arms and dumbbells back until your arms are parallel to the ground. Squeeze your triceps and return to your starting position.

③ Complete half of your repetitions with the left leg up and then switch to your right leg up. Perform this exercise for 12 to 16 repetitions.

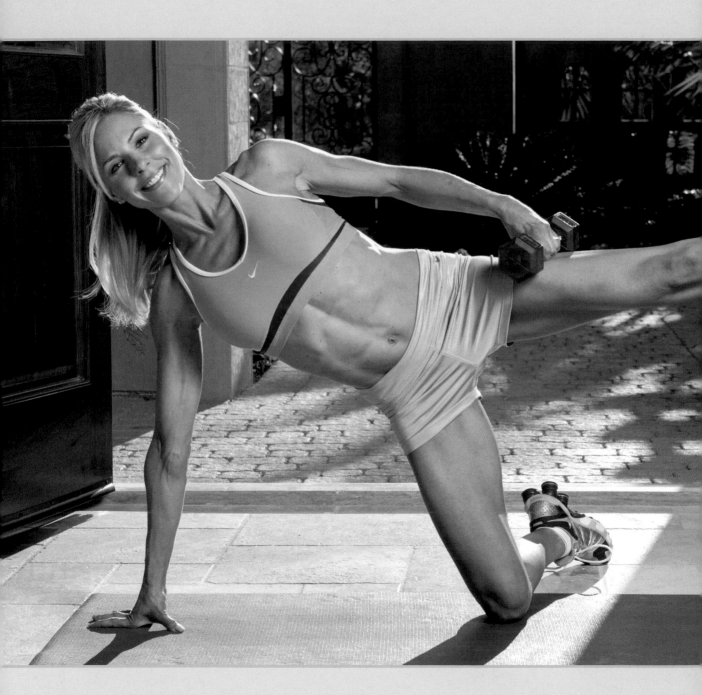

Weights for the Lower Body (Exercises 27–44)

CHAPTER 6

One topic I get a lot of questions on is how to reduce and get rid of cellulite. Clients are desperate to know why it appears, how to get rid of it, and how to prevent its horrible return. Essentially, cellulite is the buildup of fat tissue stored unevenly, which produces a dimply appearance. To speed fat loss and minimize cellulite, you must first and foremost make changes in your diet. Next, you absolutely must incorporate a combination of weight training and cardiovascular exercises in your workout routines. There's a brief but useful Ultrafit nutrition guide at the back of this book. From this guide you'll get some basic guidelines and a better understanding of the lifestyle I promote (and live every day!). If you desire a more extensive nutrition plan, visit www.ultrafitnutrition.com for more information.

Resistance training for your lower body is the key to maintaining a toned appearance (free of cellulite), and it's essential for building and keeping a high percentage of lean muscle mass versus body fat. I prefer exercises that involve a balance challenge because they force me to engage supporting muscles that might not otherwise be worked as hard (such as my core, glutes, and hip flexors). Single-leg stability leg exercises require you to engage your gluteus maximus *and* gluteus medius (a smaller muscle higher up on your hip) in order to stabilize your hips during a movement. Training these two muscles together can give you the appearance of a butt lift, and by doing these exercises regularly, you will sculpt lean muscle mass while burning excess fat at the same time!

Use the same method explained in chapter 5 to choose the amount of weight you should use for the exercises in this chapter. When you get to the last three reps, you should be fatiguing the muscle. That means that it should be difficult for you to do more than the repetitions I suggest. If I say to do twelve to fifteen reps and you can easily go to twenty, you should increase the amount of weight you are using. In chapter 13, I've designed specific workouts using all 101 exercises so that you can understand how to use the exercises in a complete workout. And as always, make sure you warm up before doing any of these exercises. (I provided some warm-up guidelines in chapter 4.) Have fun!

27 QUADS
Modified Sissy Squat (Beginner)

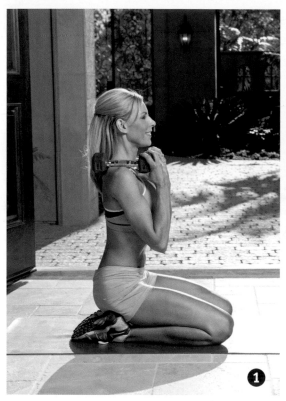

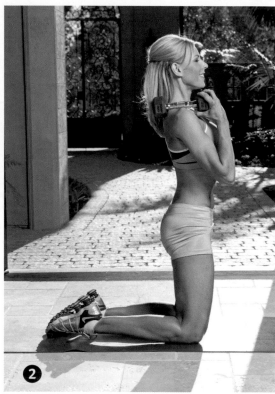

① **②**

Benefits: Strengthens quads, hips, and glutes

① Kneel on the floor, sitting back on your heels with your knees slightly apart, holding your dumbbells on your shoulders and keeping your torso erect. This is your starting position.

② Lift your hips, squeezing your glutes as you come up, while tilting your pelvis and rolling your glutes underneath your hips. Hold for 1 count, squeezing your quads and glutes, and then lower back to your starting position.

③ Repeat this exercise for 12 to 15 reps.

Seated Leg Extension (Beginner)

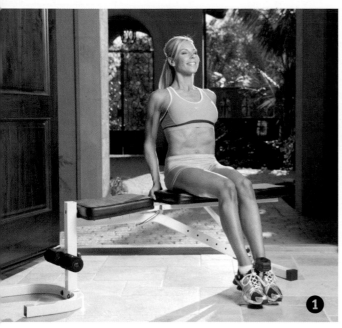 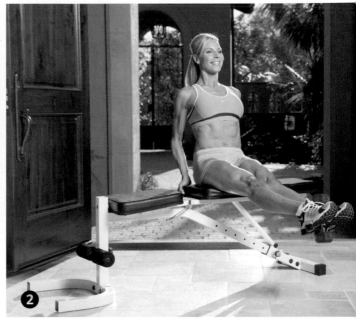

Benefit: Strengthens quads

① Sit on a bench, holding a dumbbell in between your shoes with your legs and feet together. Hold on to the bench behind you for stability. This is your starting position.

② While maintaining a tall back, extend your legs and raise the dumbbell up, squeezing your quads as you go. Slowly lower the dumbbell back down to your starting position while contracting your quads.

③ Repeat this exercise for 12 to 15 repetitions.

29

Single-Leg Bullet Squat (Advanced)

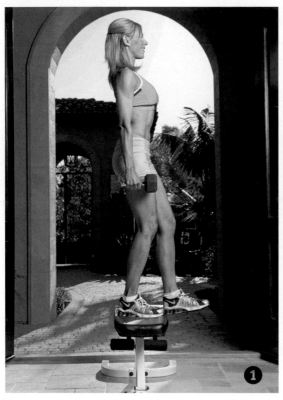

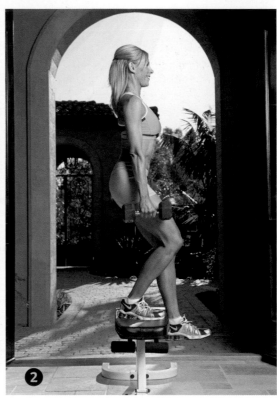

Benefits: Strengthens quads, glutes, and hamstrings

(1) Hold two dumbbells in your hands down by your sides and step up onto a bench. Extend one leg forward slightly off the bench while keeping your arms down by your sides and balancing on the other leg planted on the bench. This is your starting position.

(2) Perform your bullet squat by bending your knee, keeping the weight of your body in the heel planted on the bench as you lower your body. Squat as low as you can, but don't exceed a 90-degree angle in your knee. Return to your starting position.

(3) Repeat this exercise for 12 to 15 repetitions on each leg.

Single-Leg Step-Up (Advanced)

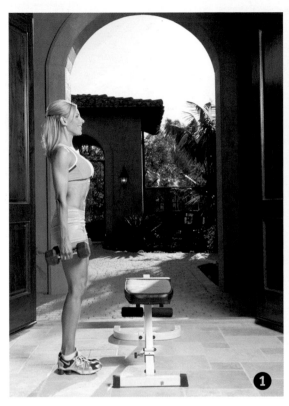 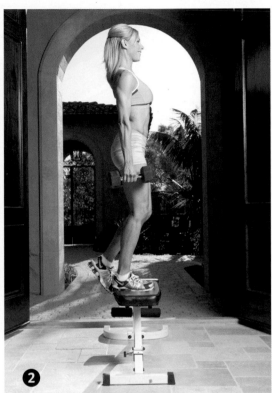

◎

Benefits: Strengthens quads, glutes, and hamstrings

① Stand while holding dumbbells, facing a flat bench or a knee-high step for your starting position.

② Put your right foot completely on top of the bench or step and use your right leg to lift your body weight. Squeeze your glutes and hamstrings tight at the top. Touch the toe of your left foot to the bench, and then slowly lower your weight back to the floor, keeping your right foot in place. Without using momentum, use your right leg to again lift your body weight.

③ Complete 12 to 15 reps on one side before switching to the other leg.

31

HAMSTRINGS
Prone Hamstring Curl (Beginner)

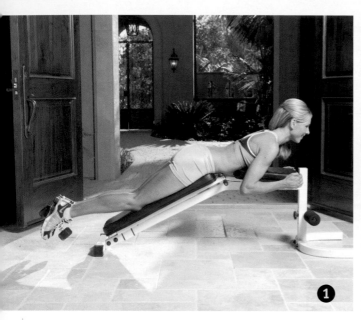 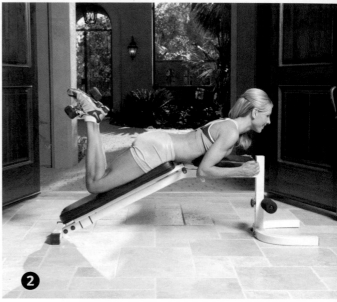

① **②**

Benefits: Strengthens hamstrings and glutes

① Lie face-down on a slightly declined bench, holding a heavier dumbbell in between your shoes tightly. Grab onto the top or sides of the bench for stability and contract your abs. This is your starting position.

② Contract your hamstrings, glutes, and abs and slowly lift the dumbbell toward your glutes (stopping before you reach your glutes), and then return back to your starting position. Try to avoid arching your back to lift the weight up.

③ Repeat this exercise for 12 to 15 repetitions.

Bridge and Scoop (Beginner)

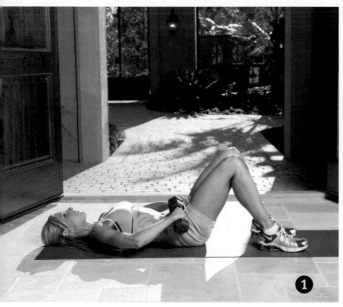

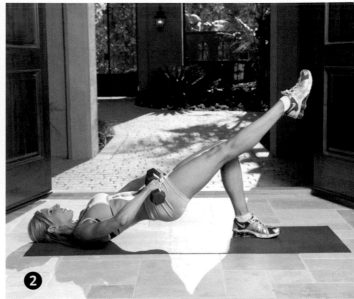

Benefits: Strengthens hamstrings and glutes

(1) Lie on your back on the floor with your knees bent at 90 degrees and your feet on the floor, with dumbbells resting on your hips. This is your starting position.

(2) Lift your hips, pull in your abs, and squeeze your glutes. Raise your right foot several inches, pointing your toes, with your knee bent. Slowly kick your leg forward and up in an arc until your leg is extended. Bend your knee, lower your leg back to the start, and repeat. Keep your hips lifted and squeeze your glutes throughout the exercise.

(3) Do all 12 to 15 reps with your right leg; lower your hips and then repeat with the opposite leg.

33

Single-Arm Cross Dead Lift (Advanced)

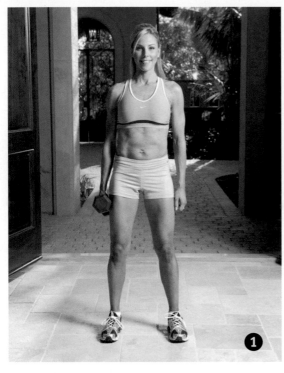 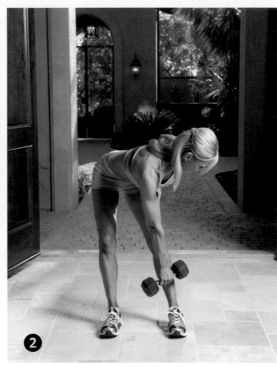

◎

Benefits: Strengthens hamstrings, glutes, and lower back

---

① Stand holding one heavier dumbbell in your right hand. Keep your abs tight and spine in a neutral position with your knees slightly bent. This is your starting position.

② Perform a single-arm cross dead lift by bending at the hips and reaching down to the outside of your left foot with your right arm. It is very important to keep your knees slightly bent, but do not squat down. Only move as far down as you can without feeling a strain in your lower back. This might be to the outside of your shin on the opposite leg. Return to the standing position.

③ Repeat for 12 to 15 repetitions on this side and then switch sides and complete the same number of reps on the other side.

Single-Leg Dead Lift (Advanced)

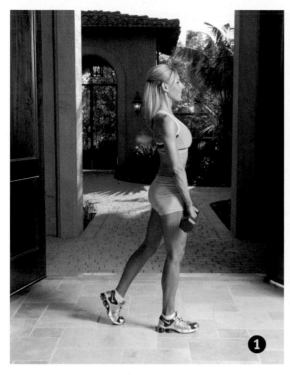 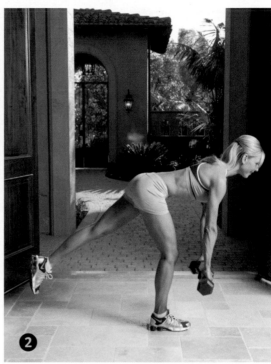

◎

Benefits: Strengthens hamstrings, glutes, and lower back

---

① Stand holding dumbbells in your hands with your arms extended down in front of your thighs. Contract your abs and maintain a neutral spine. Lift one leg up and slightly back. This is your starting position.

② Perform a single-leg dead lift by bending forward at your hips while maintain-ing a neutral spine and keeping your abs tight. Reach your dumbbells down following the line of your body until you feel a deep stretch in your hamstrings without feeling strain in your back. Keep the opposite leg up throughout the entire dead lift. Return to the standing position.

③ Complete 12 to 15 repetitions on one leg and then switch and complete the same number of repetitions on the other leg.

35

GLUTES
Reverse Lunge Torso Twist (Beginner)

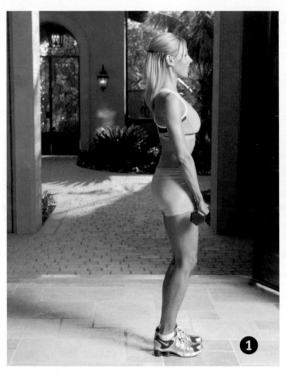

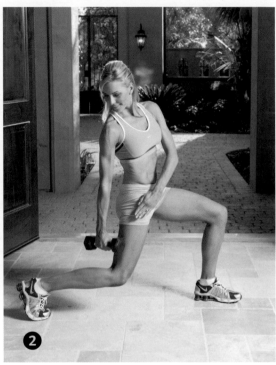

◎

Benefits: Strengthens glutes, quads, legs, and core

---

(1) Hold one dumbbell in your right hand with your arm extended down in front of your thigh and stand up straight. This is your starting position.

(2) Perform a reverse lunge by stepping back with your right leg and landing on your toes, and at the same time rotate your torso to the right by reaching your left hand across your body to the other side of your right knee. Stop the reverse lunge when your right knee is at a 90-degree angle but no deeper. Make sure to keep your body weight in the heel of the front foot. Return to the starting position by pushing off the front heel and standing back up.

(3) Complete 12 to 15 repetitions on one leg and then switch to the other leg.

Donkey Glute Kick (Beginner)

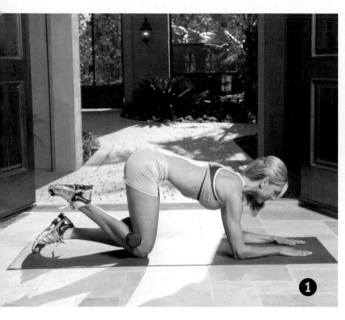 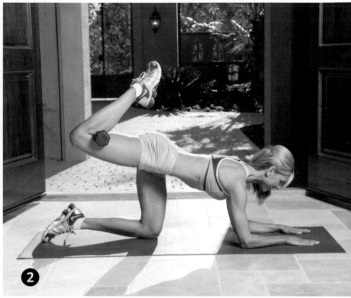

Benefits: Strengthens glutes, hamstrings, and core

① Grab one medium-weight to light dumbbell and move to the floor in a prone position on your hands and knees. Place your dumbbell at the back of one knee, lift your lower leg up, and squeeze the dumbbell between your calf and the back of your hamstring. Bend your elbows and bring them down to the floor directly under your shoulder joints. This is your starting position.

② First contract your abs, maintain a neutral spine, and lift the knee holding the dumbbell off the ground. Lead with your heel while squeezing your glutes and hamstrings until your thigh is parallel to the ground without dropping the dumbbell. Try not to arch your back or use momentum during this exercise.

③ Complete 12 to 15 repetitions on one leg and then switch to the other leg.

37

Elevated Lunge (Advanced)

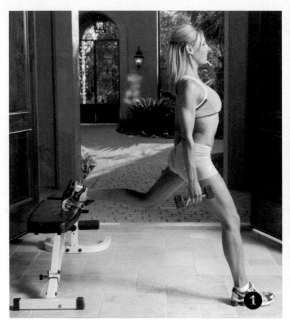 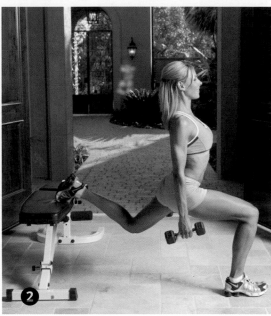

◎

Benefits: Strengthens glutes, legs, and core

① Place a flat bench about 12 to 18 inches behind you. Holding dumbbells, stand with your hands by your sides, keeping your feet about hip-width apart and toes facing forward. Step forward with one foot and lift your back leg to rest your toes on the bench behind you. Your front foot should be far enough forward so that when you're in the down position, your knee is directly in line with your heel. Keep your shoulders directly over your hips. If this is a new exercise for

you, have a spotter assist you with the setup and execution of this movement.

② Keep your torso close to vertical and the majority of your weight on your front leg as you descend into a lunge. Inhale and slowly lower your body until your front knee forms about a 90-degree angle. Push through your front heel to return to the starting position. Your forward leg should do the most work; your back leg is just for balance. Try not to lock out your knee at the top.

③ Complete 12 to 15 repetitions on one leg and then switch to the other leg.

Pulsing Diagonal Reverse Lunge and Lift (Advanced)

38

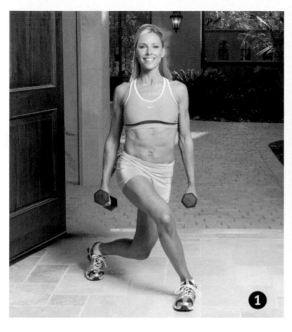

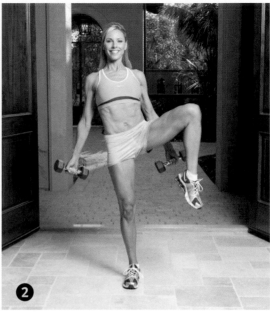

Benefits: Strengthens the glutes, hips, legs, and core

(1) Holding dumbbells, stand with your hands down by your sides. Keep your right foot and knee facing forward, as well as your entire upper body, and maintain the weight of your body in the heel of your right foot. Cross your left leg back behind you onto your toes and squat down by bending both knees. Keep your back neutral and abs tight. This is your starting position.

(2) Begin by pulsing (i.e., hold the contracting position and just move up and down about an inch) for a count of 3. (Remember to keep the weight in the heel of the front foot.) Once you are done with the pulse, push off the front heel and lift your back knee up and out to the left side while maintaining your balance, squeezing your right glute and abs. Your arms should hang down by your sides throughout the exercise.

(3) Complete 12 to 15 repetitions on one leg and then switch to the other leg.

39

Inner Thighs (Adductors)

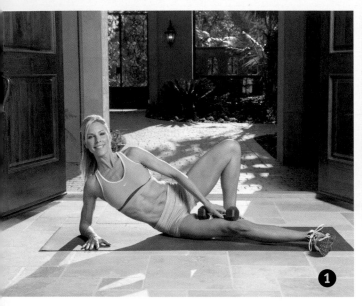

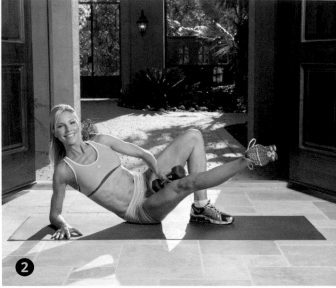

①

②

Benefits: Strengthens inner/outer thighs
---

① Grab one medium-weight dumbbell and lie on your right side on the floor. Lift your body up so you are holding your upper body by your right elbow. Slide your right leg forward and rotate your leg and foot so your toes are pointed forward. Hold a dumbbell in your left hand and place it on your right leg. Bend your left knee and place your left foot on the floor. This is your starting position.

② While holding the dumbbell on your right leg, lift your right leg up, keeping your foot parallel to the floor as you lift to engage your inner thigh. Return to the starting position.

③ Complete 12 to 15 repetitions on one leg and then switch to the other leg.

Supine Bridge Leg Extension (Intermediate/Advanced)

40

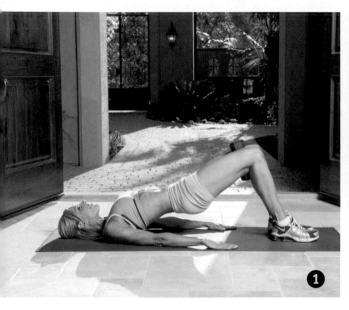

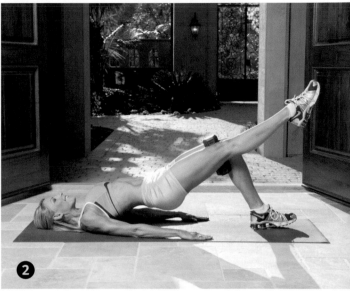

Benefits: Strengthens inner thighs, quads, glutes, hamstrings, and core

(1) Grab one medium-weight dumbbell and come to the floor in a supine bridge position by placing the dumbbell between your knees (squeezing your inner thighs to hold it). Keep your knees together and your hips raised, abs and glutes tight. This is your starting position.

(2) While holding the dumbbell between your knees, extend one leg at a time.

(3) Alternate your leg extensions, completing 12 to 15 reps on each leg.

41

OUTER THIGHS (ABDUCTORS)
Side-Plank Triangle Lift (Beginner)

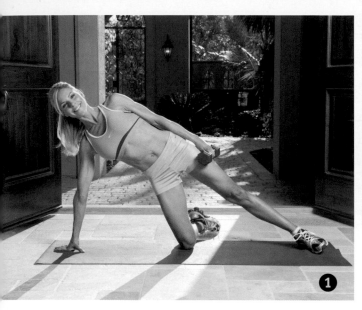

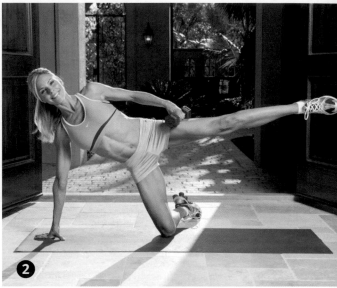

① **②**

◎

Benefits: Strengthens outer thighs and glutes

① Grab a dumbbell and kneel with your right knee on the floor. Lean to the side to place your right hand on the floor with your right palm aligned under your shoulder and your thigh perpendicular to the floor. Hold a dumbbell in your left hand and place it on your left thigh, which is extended out to the side. This is your starting position.

② Lift your left leg to hip height, with the inner thigh facing the floor and toes pointed, as you squeeze your glutes and draw in your abs. Keeping your left leg at hip height, continue to squeeze your glutes as you pull your leg 12 inches behind you. Lower your left leg until your toes are 3 to 4 inches off the floor. Lift the leg back to the starting position.

③ Complete 12 to 15 reps with your left leg and then repeat on the opposite side.

Alternating Front Curtsy Lunge (Advanced)

42

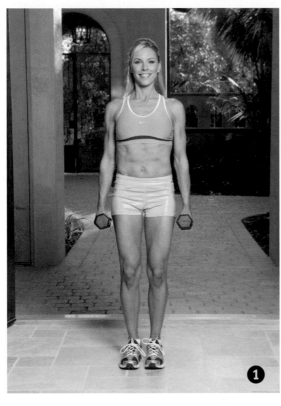

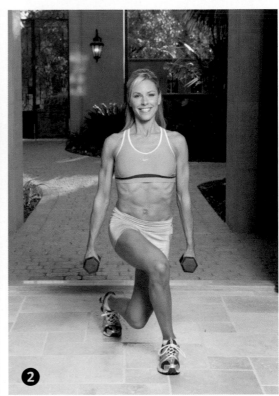

Benefits: Strengthens outer thighs, legs, and core

(1) Stand with a dumbbell in each hand with your arms down by your sides. This is your starting position.

(2) Cross your right leg in front of your left leg and bend both knees into a front curtsy lunge. Push off the heel of the front leg to return to your starting position and switch sides right away.

(3) Complete 12 to 15 repetitions on each leg, alternating legs as you go.

43

CALVES
Multi-Rep Seated Calf Raise (Beginner)

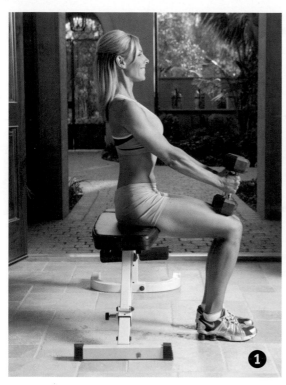 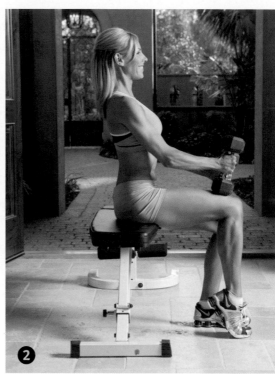

Benefit: Strengthens calves

(1) Sit on a bench, holding two heavier dumbbells on your knees, with your feet on the floor.

(2) Begin the exercise by first lifting your right heel off the floor as high as you can and squeeze your calf muscle, then lower to the ground. Next, lift your left heel up off the floor as high as you can and then lower. Then lift both heels off the floor two times. The next set you will start with your left heel, and so on. The pattern is single, single, double, double reps.

(3) Complete this exercise and cycle, single-single-double-double, 20 to 24 times. Lead with each leg 10 to 12 times.

Single-Leg Elevated Heel Raise (Intermediate)

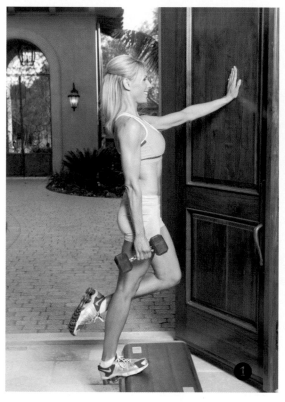
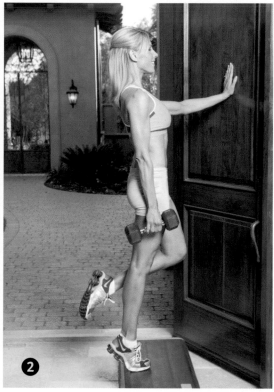

Benefit: Strengthens calves

① Hold one dumbbell in your right hand and walk to a step or an elevated area where you can hold on to something for support. Hold on with your left hand, step onto the platform, and bring your right heel off the platform and let your heel hang down. Raise your left leg. This is your starting position.

② Perform the single-leg calf raise by lifting your right heel up and squeezing your calf muscle and then return to your starting position.

③ Complete 20 to 25 repetitions on each calf.

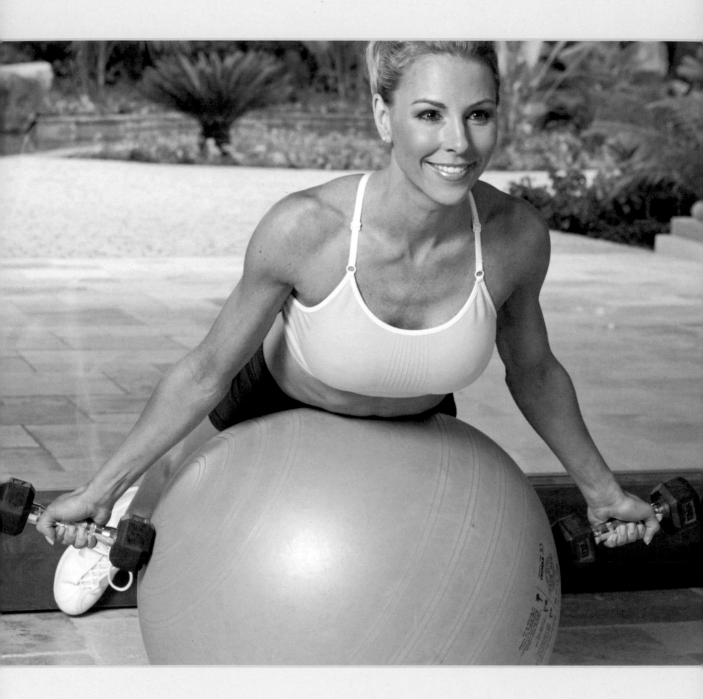

Weights on a Stability Ball
(Exercises 45–61)

T he stability ball (also known as a Swiss ball, fitness ball, physio ball, etc.) is one of the most versatile pieces of equipment available today for both home use and use in a gym setting. It was originally used primarily within the clinical rehabilitation setting, but due to its ability to help develop balance and core strength by employing multiple muscle systems, the stability ball has made the transition into the mainstream fitness community. I love the stability ball because you can actually improve joint function and joint integrity. When you are executing a movement on the stability ball, you'll discover how unstable a surface it can be. This means that your body is forced to recruit joint stabilizers and neutralizers (if you're doing the movement correctly!). All together, the stability ball will not only help get you into better shape, but it will also improve the way in which your joints function, as well as strengthen your body against possible injury. To me, there's no downside to that combination!

As a result, this chapter is dedicated to exercises with dumbbells on the stability ball. As usual, make sure you warm up (see chapter 4). Have fun!

45

BACK
Stability Ball Upper-Back Pump (All Levels)

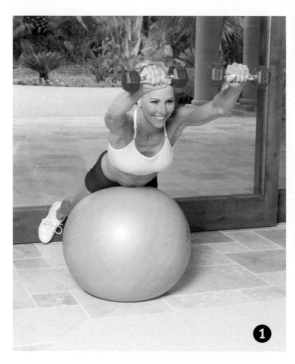

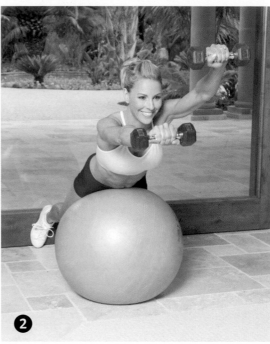

Benefits: Works upper and lower back,
core, and shoulders

---

① Start on your knees with the stability
ball in front of you. Roll yourself onto
the ball until your lower abdominals and
hips are supported and brace the soles
of your shoes against a wall for support.
Holding a light dumbbell (1 to 3
pounds) in each hand, lift your chest
(look forward/down in order to keep
your neck in neutral alignment with
your spine) and straighten and extend
your arms forward, keeping them
close to your ears. This is your
starting position.

② Pulse your arms up and down (2 to
3 inches).

③ Repeat the movement for 12 to
15 repetitions.

Hyperextension (All Levels)

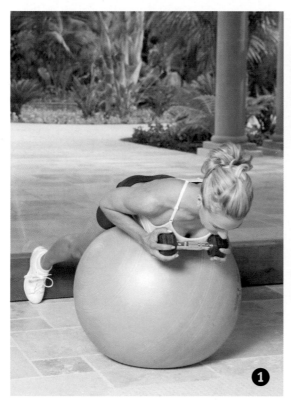
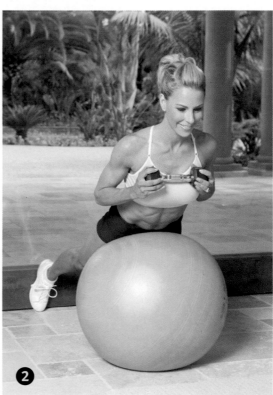

1
2

Benefits: Works upper and lower back, core, and shoulders

① Start on your knees with the stability ball in front of you. Roll yourself onto the ball until your lower abdominals and hips are supported and brace the soles of your shoes against a wall for support. Hold a single dumbbell with both hands

against your chest. This is your starting position.

② Raise your upper body until your knees, hips, and shoulders are all in line. Lower your upper body back down to the ball.

③ Repeat the movement for 12 to 15 repetitions.

47

CHEST
Supine Bridge Chest Press (All Levels)

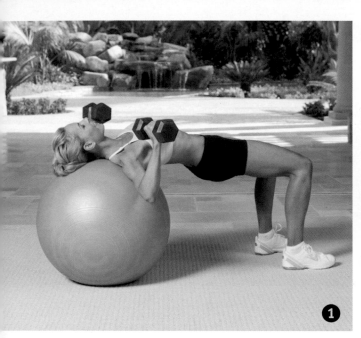

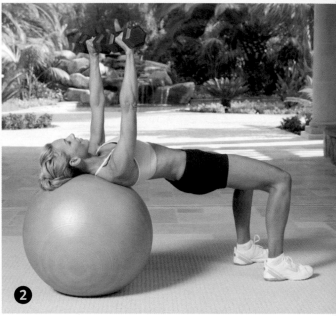

①   **②**

◎

Benefits: Works pectorals, core, biceps

① Start in a seated position on the stability ball, holding the weights you will be pressing in each hand. From this seated position, slowly roll yourself out until your neck and shoulders are supported by the ball. Your feet should be positioned slightly wider than hip-width apart, and your knees are bent. Contract your abdominals and lift your hips until your body is in a flat "bridge" position.

Your weights should be positioned on either side of your chest and your palms facing forward. This is your starting position.

② Press your arms upward, extending the weights directly above your sternum. Once you have reached the top, hold the extension and contract your pectorals, and then slowly bring the weights back to the starting position.

③ Repeat the movement for 12 to 15 repetitions.

Alternating Chest Fly, One Leg Up (Intermediate/Advanced)

48

---◎---

Benefits: Works pectorals, core, biceps

① Start in a seated position on the stability ball, holding the weights you will be using in each hand. From this seated position, slowly roll yourself out until your neck and shoulders are supported by the ball. Contract your abdominals and lift your hips until your body is in a flat "bridge" position. Position one foot slightly off-center, and lift and extend the opposite leg off the ground. Extend your arms up directly above your shoulders, keeping your elbows slightly bent. This is your starting position.

② Alternating arms, move the dumbbell in a horizontal plane across your body.

③ Repeat the movement for 6 to 8 repetitions with the left leg elevated, and 6 to 8 repetitions with the right leg elevated.

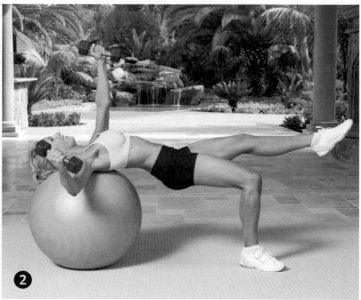

❶

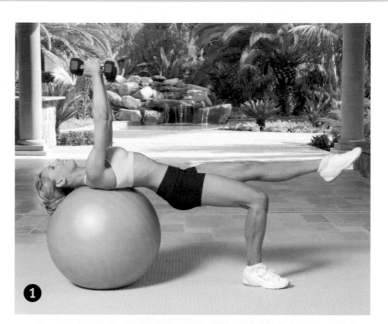

❷

49

SHOULDERS
Stability Ball Cobra
(Beginner/Intermediate)

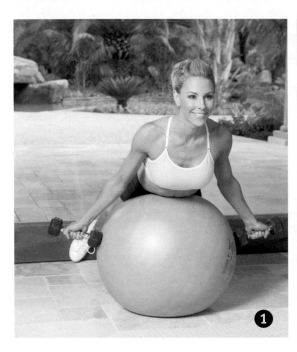

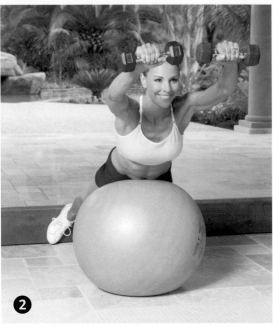

◎

Benefits: Works middle and lower traps, lats, internal and external rotators, glutes, and spinal stabilizers

① Hold two lighter dumbbells in both hands and kneel on the floor with the stability ball in front of you. Roll yourself onto the ball until your lower abdominals and hips are supported and brace the soles of your shoes against a wall for support. Lift your chest (look forward/down in order to keep your neck in neutral alignment with your spine) and straighten and extend your arms back toward your glutes with your palms facing down. This is your starting position.

② Squeeze your shoulder blades together and bring your arms out to the sides and forward over your head, rotating your arms so that your palms are down and directly over your head. Pinch your shoulders together and arch your back in order to hold the pose. Then take your arms back to your starting position.

③ Repeat the movement for 12 to 15 repetitions.

Alternating Overhead Extensions, One Leg Up (Intermediate/Advanced)

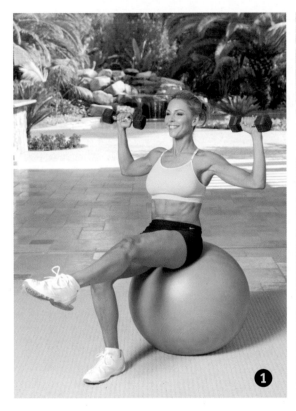
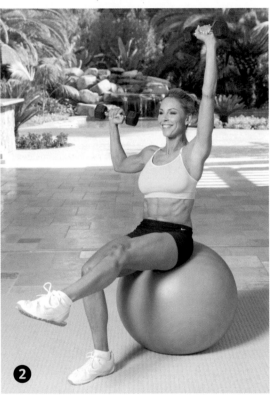

1 **2**

◎

Benefits: Works shoulders, lats, quads

(1) Start in a seated position on the stability ball, holding the weights you will be using in each hand. Position one foot slightly off-center, and lift and extend the opposite leg off the ground. Bring your upper arms up to shoulder level,

and bend your elbows so that your forearms are vertical. This is your starting position.

(2) Alternating arms, extend each arm and push the dumbbell overhead.

(3) Repeat the movement for 6 to 8 repetitions with the left leg elevated, and 6 to 8 repetitions with the right leg elevated.

51

QUADS/BICEPS
Stability Ball Wall Squats with Biceps Curl (Beginner)

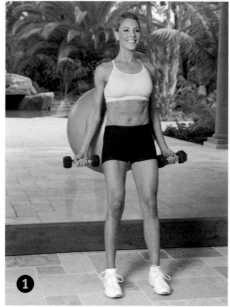

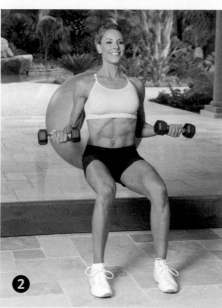

Benefits: Works quads, glutes, hamstrings, biceps, and core

(1) Start by standing away from a wall. Place a stability ball against the wall at lower-back height and squeeze it against the wall with your lower back. Your feet should be shoulder-width apart with toes pointing forward, approximately 10 to 12 inches in front of your body. Hold a dumbbell in each hand, at your sides. This is your starting position.

(2) Pressing into the ball, sit into a squatting position by lowering your body until your knees are flexed at 90-degree angles. Make sure that your knees do not pass over your toes, and that you press your weight through your heels. As you move into the sitting position, bend your elbows and curl the weights toward your biceps. Extend your legs to move back into a standing position, while at the same time lowering the weights back to your sides.

(3) Repeat the movement for 12 to 15 repetitions.

BICEPS
Stability Ball Preacher Curl (Beginner)

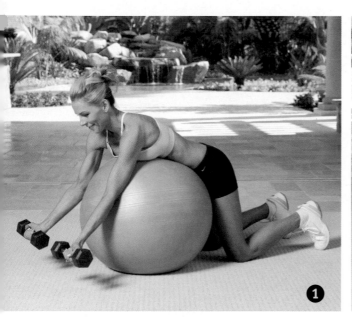 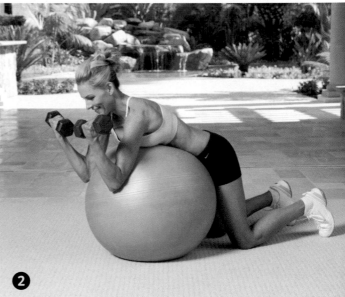

1 **2**

◎

Benefits: Works biceps

① This is a standard biceps curl using the stability ball. Start in a kneeling position facing a stability ball. Hold a dumbbell in each hand, and stabilize your elbows by leaning your upper body over the ball and pressing your elbows into it. Your arms should be extended. This is your starting position.

② Bend your elbows, bring the weights towards your shoulders, and contract your biceps.

③ Repeat the movement for 12 to 15 repetitions.

53

TRICEPS
Elevated Triceps Dips (Advanced)

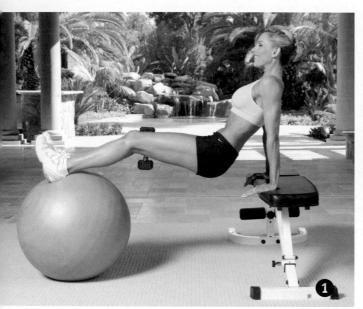

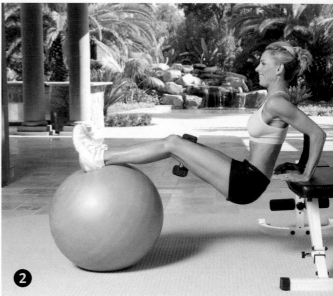

Benefits: Works triceps

(1) Place your hands on the edge of a bench, extend your legs, elevate your feet on a stability ball, and grip a single dumbbell between your thighs. This is your starting position.

(2) Keep your elbows tight to the sides of your body as you lower your body toward the floor, and use your triceps to push yourself back up. Do not lock out your elbows at the top of the movement.

(3) Repeat the movement for 12 to 15 repetitions.

ABDOMINALS
Supine Gator Rotation (Advanced)

54

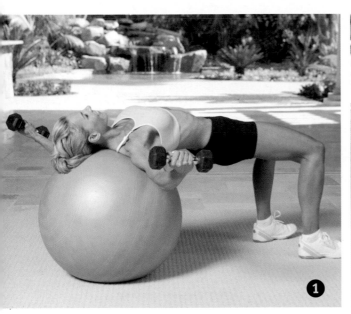

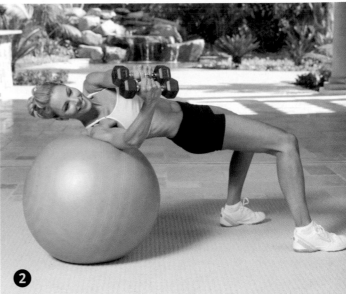

① **②**

◎

Benefit: Works core

---

① Start in a seated position on a stability ball, holding the weights you will be using in each hand. From this seated position, lie back until your upper and middle back are supported by the ball. Hold the weights at chest level and then extend your arms out laterally to your sides, with your elbows bent. This is your starting position.

② Keeping your abs tight and your arms straight and elbows slightly bent, take one weight and touch it to the other while rotating your torso (side-to-side). Your arms should move together like the jaws of an alligator snapping shut.

③ Repeat the movement for 12 to 15 repetitions.

55

Long-Lever Trunk Curl (Beginner)

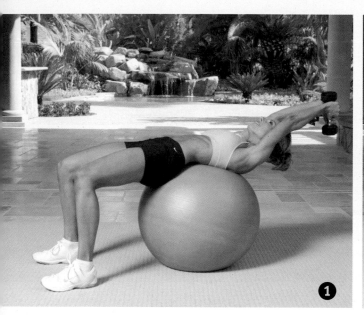

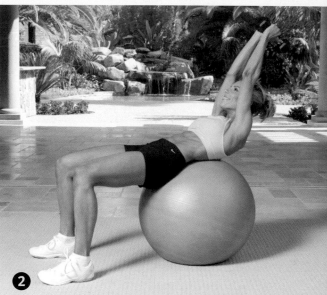

◎

Benefit: Works core

① Start in a seated position on the stability ball, holding a single dumbbell with both hands. Slowly roll down, keeping your abdominals tight, until your lower back is supported by the ball. From here, extend your arms back and over your head, holding the dumbbell with straight arms over your head. This is your starting position.

② Tighten your abdominals, and raise your torso, arms, and upper back all at the same time, contracting your abs while keeping your arms and elbows close to your ears. Hold the contraction at the peak for a pause and then return to your starting position.

③ Repeat the movement for 12 to 15 repetitions.

Crunch with Rotation (All Levels)

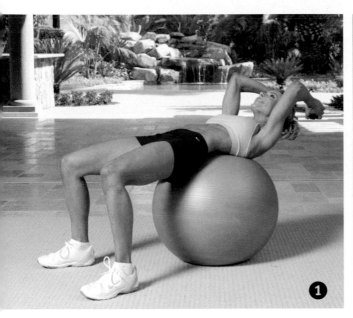

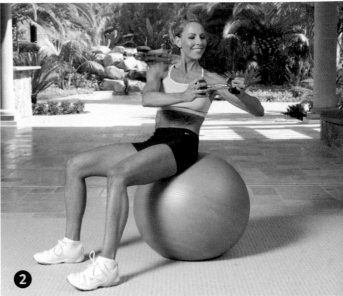

Benefit: Works core

① Start in a seated position on the stability ball, holding a single dumbbell with both hands at your chest. Slowly roll down, keeping your abdominals tight, until your lower back is supported by the ball. Bend your elbows and bring your arms and the dumbbell behind your head. This is your starting position.

② Tightening your abdominals, roll up and "crunch" by raising your shoulders and upper back in toward your hips, and rotate your torso to one side. Lower your torso, and repeat the movement with rotation to the opposite side.

③ Repeat the full movement (rotation to each side) for 12 to 15 repetitions.

57 Oblique Cross Chop (All Levels)

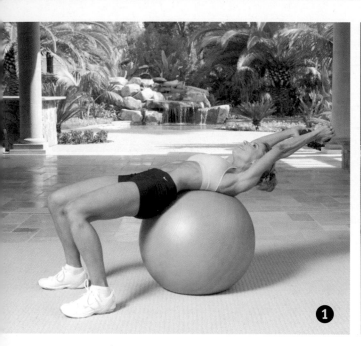

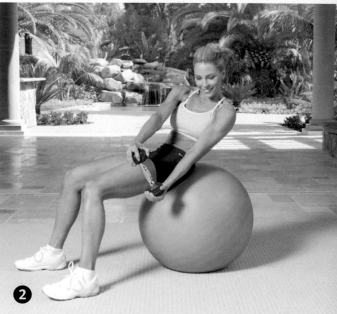

1 **2**

Benefit: Works core

(1) Start in a seated position on the stability ball, holding a single dumbbell with both hands. Slowly roll down, keeping your abdominals tight, until your lower back is supported by the ball. Reach the dumbbell and your arms back into a long stretch over your head. This is your starting position.

(2) Pull your abs in and roll up, moving your arms and the dumbbell in a diagonal direction to the opposite thigh with a wood chopping–like action. Return to your starting position.

(3) Repeat the movement, alternating from side to side, for 12 to 15 repetitions on each side.

GLUTES/HAMSTRINGS
Hip Raise (Beginner)

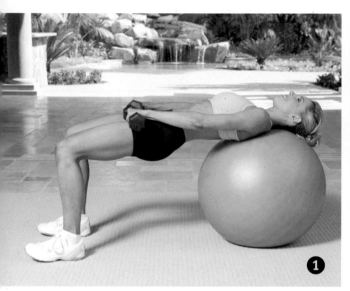
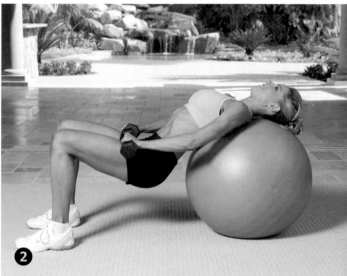

Benefits: Works glutes, hamstrings, and lower back

(1) Start in a seated position on a stability ball, holding two dumbbells in your hands, and slowly roll yourself out until your head and shoulders are supported by the ball. Your feet should be positioned slightly wider than hip-width apart, and your knees are bent. Contract your abdominals and lift your hips until your body is in a flat "bridge" position. Place your dumbbells on your thighs. This is your starting position.

(2) Lower your hips towards the ground, and then squeeze your glutes to bring them back up to the "bridge" position.

(3) Repeat the movement for 12 to 15 repetitions.

59 Reverse Rolling Single-Leg Lunge (Advanced)

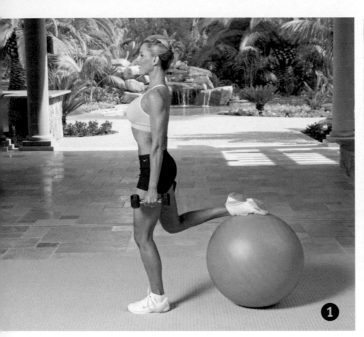 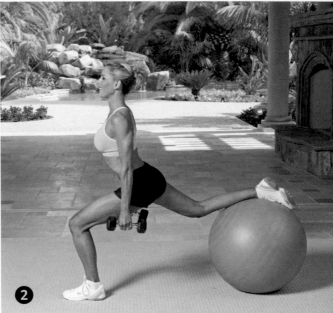

Benefits: Works quads, hamstrings, glutes, and hip flexors

---

① Stand in front of a stability ball holding dumbbells in your hands by your sides. Place the top of your right foot on top of the ball. Bring your left foot forward and make sure you press your weight through the heel of this support leg. The toes of the support leg should be pointing forward. This is your starting position.

② Keeping your shoulders back and your abdominals tight to avoid torso sway, drop your hips and roll your right leg back on the stability ball until the support leg is flexed 90 degrees. The knee should track straight over the ankle. Press through the heel and extend the support leg to raise your body back into standing.

③ Repeat the movement on your right side for 12 to 15 repetitions, then switch to your left side for 12 to 15 repetitions.

Forward Sliding Single-Leg Squat (Advanced)

60

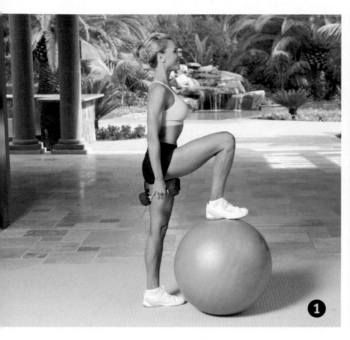

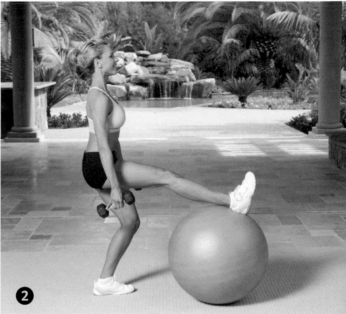

◎

Benefits: Works quads and inner and outer thighs

① Stand next to your stability ball holding dumbbells in your hands by your sides. Place your right foot on top of the ball, and plant your left. This is your starting position.

② Make sure to contract your abdominals to avoid torso sway and sit into a single-leg squat by lowering your body as deep as you can on your left leg, making sure the left knee doesn't go beyond the toe. At the same time, press your right foot into the top of the ball and roll it away from your body. As you press through the heel of the left foot to stand by extending the left leg, roll the ball toward you.

③ Repeat the movement on your right side for 12 to 15 repetitions, then switch to your left side for 12 to 15 repetitions.

61

CALVES
Toe Calf Running (Beginner)

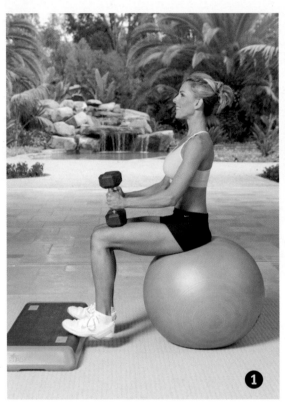

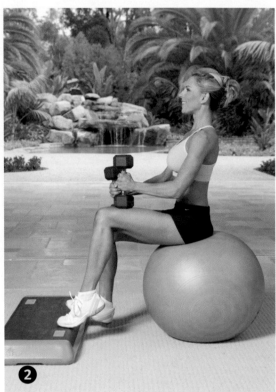

Benefits: Works calves and core

① Sit tall on a stability ball with your knees bent 90 degrees. Hold dumbbells on your thighs and rest the balls of your feet on a raised platform. This is your starting position.

② Drawing your abs in, lift and lower your heels, alternating feet.

③ Repeat the movement for 12 to 15 repetitions.

Weights for Cardio and Plyometric Training (Exercises 62–66)

CHAPTER 8

One of the best ways to maximize fat loss and get more out of your aerobic training is to vary both the duration and intensity of your cardio workouts by incorporating plyometric moves. These are moves that require a person to quickly transfer power, balance, and energy (so that the move is often "explosive"). These plyometric moves allow the body to gain muscle, improve athletic endurance, burn extra calories, and help you get over those nasty fitness plateaus that sometimes get us down.

For two of the exercises in this chapter, you will need a space that's large enough to run in. The first is the Dumbbell Run, and the second is the Lateral Shuffling Dumbbell Switch. Here in San Diego, I like to take my Ultrafit clients to the beach for a boot camp–like workout where I do all kinds of cardio and plyometric training–type exercises. The sand is a great place to do this because the softer and uneven surface makes it more difficult to keep your balance during the exercise, thus forcing your body to recruit more muscle fibers to keep upright. The more muscles you work, the more calories you burn, and the leaner and fitter your body will become! Now I know what you are thinking—not everyone lives by the ocean. Being from North Dakota, I certainly understand where you're coming from! The next best place is a big grassy area or park.

Review what I wrote about proper form and alignment in chapter 2; it's especially important here. Keep your weight over the center of your body when appropriate for the exercise, stand tall with your shoulders back and down (relaxed, not tense), pull your rib cage in—don't extend it—and pull in your tummy tight. Your pelvis needs to be in a neutral alignment (your tailbone should be pointing down), and your abdominals should be contracted with the rib cage down. Remember, correctly contracting your abdominal area (pulling your belly button in towards your spine) should not impede your ability to breathe in any way. The parameters for the amount of weight to be used are the same here as they were for chapters 5 and 6.

See chapter 13 for some more specific workouts using all 101 exercises you can use for a complete workout. See chapter 4 for some suggested warm-up exercises. These plyometric exercises are different and challenging, so have fun!

62

Dumbbell Run (Advanced)

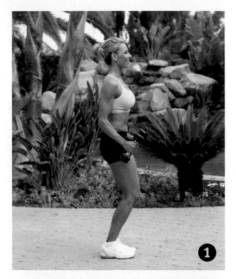

Benefits: Strengthens cardiovascular system, improves leg strength, and burns calories and fat

1. Begin by holding light to medium dumbbells in your hands, with your arms down by your sides and your elbows slightly bent.

1. Start with a slow jog and increase your speed so that you're running as fast as you can to your ending point. Your arms and dumbbells may swing naturally or stay at your sides. Your ending point will be determined by your ability. If you are just starting out, you might just jog for a short distance and then pick it up as you get stronger.

1. Return to your starting position and do it again for 15 to 20 repetitions, depending on your ability and goals.

Note: You will need at least 30 yards (27 meters) to make this exercise effective.

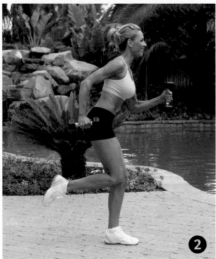

Plié Pop-Up
(Beginner/Intermediate)

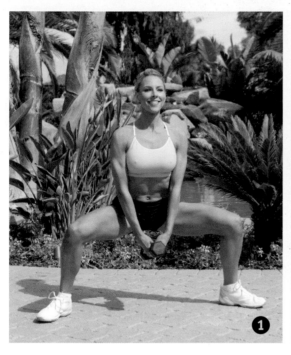

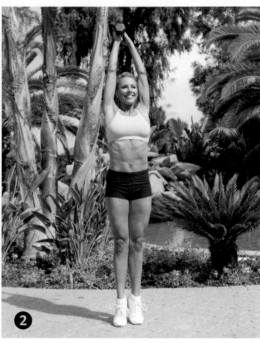

◎

Benefits: Strengthens hamstrings, quads,
glutes, core, and shoulders

① Hold one dumbbell in both hands with
your arms extended down in front of
your body and your legs in a plié position, with your knees bent. Your feet
should be wider than shoulder-width
apart and your toes turned outward, with
your back straight.

② Keeping your shoulders aligned directly
above your hips and your weight in the
center of your body (don't shift weight
from side to side), jump your feet
together while contracting your stomach
and butt muscles. At the same time,
raise your arms and swing the dumbbell
up and over your head; you should feel
a stretch through the center of your abs.
Pause here and return to the starting
position.

③ Complete the exercise for 12 to 15
repetitions.

64 Lateral Shuffling Dumbbell Switch (Beginner/Intermediate)

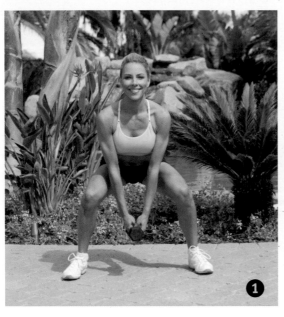

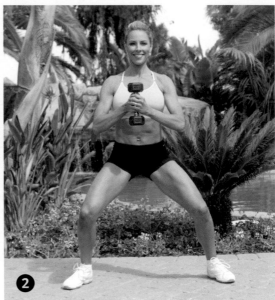

Benefits: Strengthens cardiovascular system, legs, and core

(1) Place two dumbbells down on the ground at least 20 feet apart. Beginning at dumbbell #1, squat down, keeping your head up, chest up, and glutes down. Pick up dumbbell #1 and hold it in both hands.

(2) Bring dumbbell #1 close to your stomach and side shuffle by stepping your feet (step together, step together) until you're at dumbbell #2. Squat down again, placing dumbbell #1 on the

ground and picking up dumbbell #2. Side shuffle back to the starting position, squat down again, and place dumbbell #2 on the ground. Leave dumbbell #2 there and side shuffle back to dumbbell #1. Squat down, pick up dumbbell #1, and side shuffle back to dumbbell #2. This is one repetition.

(3) Repeat this exercise for 10 to 20 repetitions, or whatever your ability will allow.

Note: You will need a 20-foot space for this exercise.

Single-Arm Power Clean (Advanced)

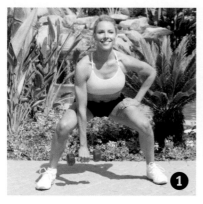

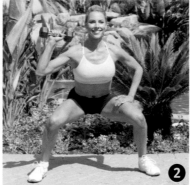

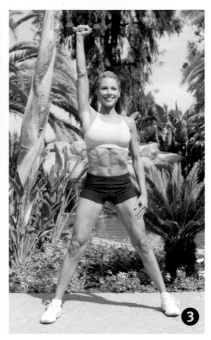

Benefits: Strengthens legs, core, and upper body

① Hold one medium-weight dumbbell in your right hand with your arm extended down and your palm facing your body. Step your legs wider than hip-width apart, maintain a tall back and tight abs, and squat down like a sumo wrestler, so your thighs are parallel to the ground, your chest and head up, and your glutes down. This is your starting position.

② Explode in an upward motion, lifting your feet off the ground by a few inches while lifting your arm and dumbbell to shoulder height; land back down in a squat position with your dumbbell by your shoulder.

③ From this position, stand up by pushing off on your heels and perform a one-arm overhead shoulder press. Bring the dumbbell back down to your shoulder again.

④ Return the dumbbell and your body back down to your starting position, pause in the squat, and repeat the exercise, not stopping for 12 to 15 repetitions. Repeat the exercise for 12 to 15 repetitions holding the dumbbell in your left hand.

66 Squat and Jump Shoulder Press (Advanced)

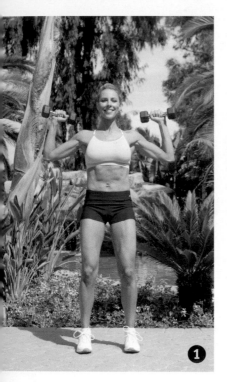
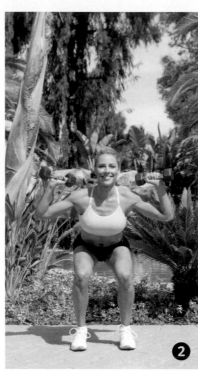
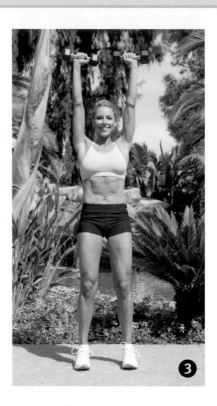

Benefits: Strengthens legs, shoulders, and core

---

(1) Stand with a dumbbell in each hand at chin level. Face straight ahead with your ab muscles tight.

(2) Lower to a full squat position with your knees at a 90-degree angle but no lower. Keep your weight centered between the balls of your feet and your heels. Keep your shoulders, hips, and ankles in a vertical line.

(3) Follow the squat with an explosive jump into a jumping overhead shoulder press movement, done in one fluid motion, and landing with your knees softly bent.

(4) Return to your starting position and repeat for 12 to 15 repetitions.

Weights for Core Training and Postural Improvement (Exercises 67–80)

CHAPTER 9

"Stand up straight!" "Pull your shoulders back!" "Hold your stomach in!" Do any of these orders sound familiar? Having good posture does more than make your mother happy. Improving your posture has a direct impact on your physical and mental well-being, as well as your self-esteem. One of the best ways to maintain proper posture and stabilization is to strengthen your chest, back, and core muscles with strength training.

✳ Preventing Back Pain

Posture training and core training are a huge part of my workouts because I personally deal with my own degenerative lower-back condition. My L-5 and L-4 vertebrae compress my SI joint, causing lower-back pain, as well as shooting pains down my left leg. It's a hereditary condition, so my family members have dealt with it for years. I've seen a lot of methods for relieving the pain, but so far, the training I do has been the only way I've been able to help prevent problems and maintain a relatively pain-free body. The only reason I am able to continue to train and work out the way I do is because of the strength training, core training, and posture exercises I incorporate into my workouts on a regular basis. That is why this chapter is so very important to me.

The Mayo Clinic recently reported that four out of five adults experience at least one bout of back pain at some point during their lifetimes. The Mayo researchers found that back injuries are the leading cause of work-related disability. The causes of lower-back pain are numerous—injuries, muscle strains, muscle spasms, joint disorders, herniated disks, and the list goes on. Not all back injuries are completely preventable, but there are some ways to reduce the overall incidence and severity of back pain. Through my research, I've come up with the following tips for preventing lower-back pain:

Don't lift by bending over. Instead, bend your hips and knees and then squat to pick up your item. Keep your back straight and hold the object close to your body. Always avoid twisting while lifting as well.

✔ Push heavy objects instead of pulling them.

✔ Try not to sit for long periods of time without getting up or stretching. Try to get up and stretch every 30 to 40 minutes.

✔ Exercise regularly! Inactivity contributes to lower-back pain. Focus on my core and posture exercises when you are planning your workouts!

✔ Try to use chairs with straight backs or with lower-back support. Keep your knees at hip height or slightly higher.

✔ If you have to stand for long periods, rest one foot on a low stool to reduce the pressure on your spine, then switch feet every 15 minutes or so.

✔ Practice good posture by pulling in your abs, sitting up straight, and pulling your shoulders back during normal daily activities like standing in line, sitting, or driving. The more you hold that posture, the stronger you will be!

The Correct Way to Perform a Sit-Up

I see so many people in the gym day in and day out doing sit-ups the incorrect way. Powering through their hip flexors, cranking on their necks, and incorrect breathing are all pretty common mistakes. When performed properly, sit-ups help tone the muscles in your midsection, which can help protect your back as well as add to your desired "six-pack" appearance. When done incorrectly, however, sit-ups can be a waste of time and possibly even harmful.

It doesn't matter what kind of sit-up you are doing or even if you're doing another type of core movement that requires you to tighten your abs. Your first step should be to slow down your movement, as if you are in slow motion. Focus on using your abdominal muscles only. Close your eyes and visualize the abdominal muscles tensing and shortening like a shoe string that draws your shoulders and head off the floor. Your second step should be to exhale while the abdominal muscles contract and pull you upward. This will pull the muscles inward, requiring the involvement of the deeper abdominal muscles.

Inhaling will cause your abdomen to protrude (causing a bulge), and may lead to over-arching and straining of your lower back. Third, bending your knees during sit-ups helps neutralize the action of the hip flexors and makes the abdominal muscles work more. You will find that while doing any kind of straight-leg sit-up, you will feel your hip flexors tighten as you utilize them during the movement. The straight-leg version may also be hazardous to your lower back if you are not careful because of the extreme lower-back arch it usually creates. And lastly, make sure that when doing any type of sit-up, you stop immediately at the slightest pain in your lower back.

✳ Abdominal Newsflash!

Although I love working my abs and core, and using posture exercises to improve my midsection, strengthening your abs will *not* remove fat from the waistline. There is no such thing as spot reduction, because muscles do not fuel exercise by using the fat that surrounds them. Instead, during exercise the body tends to mobilize fat from storage depots throughout the body, so the fat used as fuel during sit-ups may come from the legs, back, face, or other areas. To remove body fat, you must burn calories. The abdominal muscle group is relatively small, and the number of calories expended during a couple of sit-ups is minimal. To truly see a six-pack in your midsection (or to just have a flat stomach), you must do core training along with a combination of cardiovascular exercise and modified nutrition. Check out chapter 14 for my Ultrafit nutrition guide!

67

ABS/CORE/POSTURE
Frog-Legs Ab Crunch (Beginner)

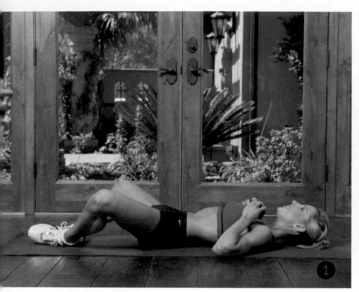 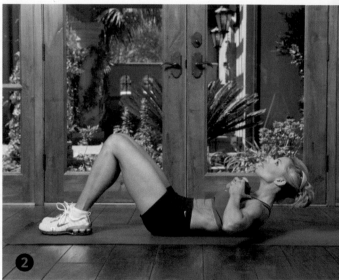

◎

Benefits: Strengthens abdominals and inner thighs

① Grab one light to medium-weight dumbbell, lie down on the floor, and hold it to your chest. Let your knees fall down to the sides in a bent froglike position. This is your starting position.

② Contract your abs by pulling in your belly button, and lift your head slightly from the floor. Lift your shoulder blades off the floor, exhaling as you lift, while at the same time lifting your knees by squeezing your inner thighs and bringing them together at the top of your contraction. Then bring your upper body and knees back down at the same time.

③ Repeat the exercise for 20 to 30 repetitions.

Frontal Plane Oblique Side Bend (Beginner)

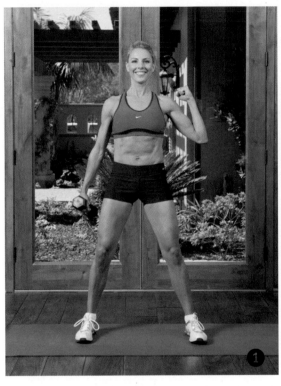
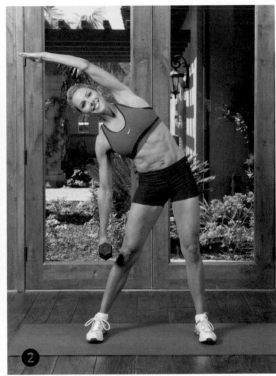

Benefits: Strengthens oblique ab muscles and core

1. Begin by standing with your feet just wider than shoulder-width apart, holding one medium-weight to heavy dumbbell in your right hand down by your side, and your left arm bent with your hand outside of your shoulder.

2. Perform the side bend by first contracting your abs and slightly tilting your pelvis forward. Bend your body sideways in the frontal plane while reaching your left arm up over your head and toward the right side. The dumbbell will follow along your side as you bend.

3. Come back to your starting position. Complete the exercise for 12 to 15 repetitions on each side.

69 Bent-Over Rear Delt into Back Rows (Beginner)

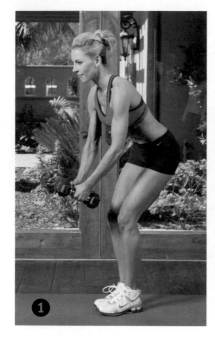
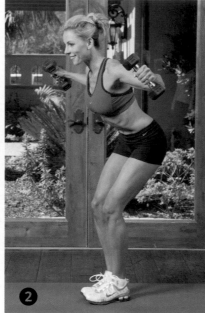
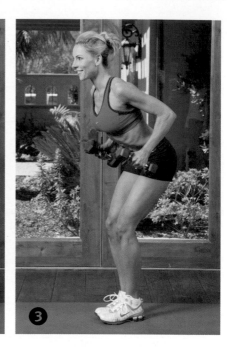

Benefits: Strengthens posterior deltoids, lats, and rhomboids

① Hold a light to medium-weight dumbbell in each hand. From a standing position, lean over with your spine either at a 45-degree angle to or parallel with (the more advanced version) the floor and arms hanging down toward the ground, with your palms facing each other. This is your starting position.

② Start the move by lifting the dumbbells up and out laterally, just like you are spreading your wings. Contract your rhomboids and return to your starting position.

③ For the second part of this exercise, maintain your spine either at a 45-degree angle to or parallel with the floor. Then bring the dumbbells toward your body and pull your elbows up and back for the back row. Your elbows should form right angles at the completion of the movement. Squeeze your back and return to the starting position.

④ Perform the exercise for 12 to 15 repetitions.

Bent-Over Row with Supinated Wrists (Beginner)

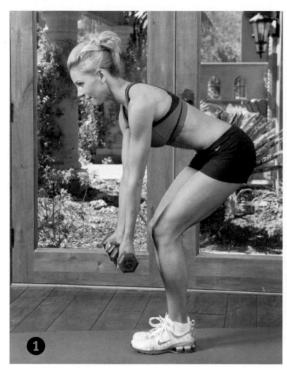

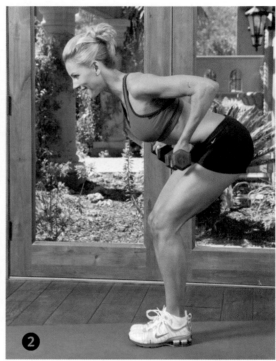

Benefits: Strengthens rhomboids, lats, and biceps

① Grab two medium-weight dumbbells. Lean over with your spine either at a 45-degree angle to or parallel with (the more advanced version) the floor and arms hanging down toward the ground, with your palms facing away from your body (supinated wrists). This is your starting position.

② Maintain your spine position. Then pull both dumbbells up to your sides for one back row. Your elbows should form right angles at the completion of the movement. Squeeze your back and return to the starting position.

③ Perform the exercise for 12 to 15 repetitions.

71 Half Sit-Up (Beginner)

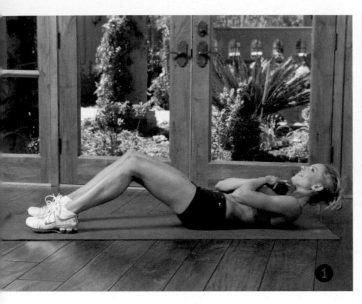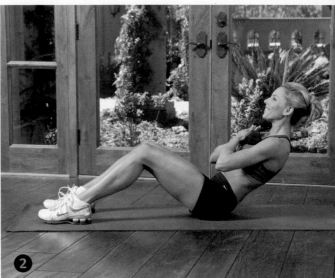

Benefits: Strengthens rectus abdominis and hip flexors

① Holding a light to medium-weight dumbbell, lie down and cross your arms over your chest. Keep your knees bent. If you'd like, hook your feet under something stable at floor level, such as a couch or heavy chair. This is your starting position.

② Perform a sit-up only halfway up and pause. Continue all the way up.

③ Lower back to the halfway position, then pause again and lower all the way. That's one rep. Perform 25 to 50 reps.

Prone Rear Deltoid Raise (Beginner)

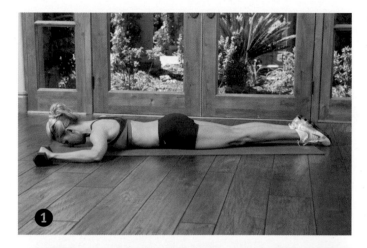

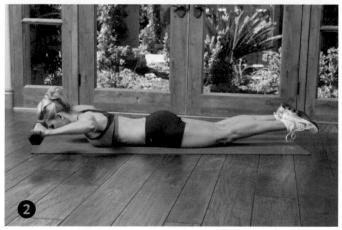

Benefits: Strengthens rear delts
and rhomboids

1. Lie on the floor with your arms out to your sides. Your elbows are bent at 90-degree angles. This is your starting position.

2. Raise your dumbbells and elbows up while squeezing your shoulder blades together. Keep your fore-arms parallel to the floor, and at the same time lift your feet off the ground only a couple of inches, squeezing your glutes and lower back. Your neck should stay neutral and your head should face down.

3. Return to your starting position.

4. Perform the exercise for 12 to 15 repetitions.

73 Side Oblique Dumbbell Rotation (Advanced)

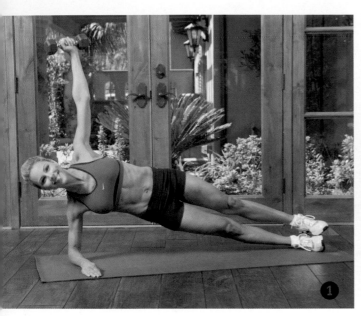

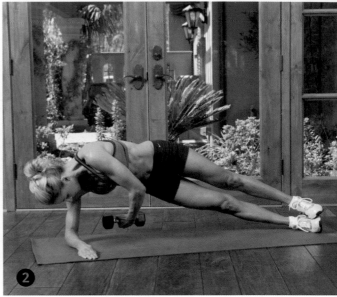

Benefits: Strengthens oblique abdominal muscles, shoulders, and core

(1) Grab a light to medium-weight dumbbell and come to the floor in a side plank position, with your upper body supported by your elbow, your hips up, and your feet stacked on top of each other. (To make it less advanced, you may do this exercise with no weight or with your bottom knee bent and on the floor for support.) Push your top arm straight up, holding the dumbbell in your hand. This is your starting position.

(2) Hold your side plank position, exhale, and bring the dumbbell down and under your body, contracting your abs and oblique muscles. Make sure to stay tight in your core, do not sink into your shoulder, and keep your hips up.

(3) Bring the dumbbell back up to your starting position. Repeat the exercise for 12 to 15 repetitions on each side.

Balancing Single-Leg Bent-Over Row (Advanced)

74

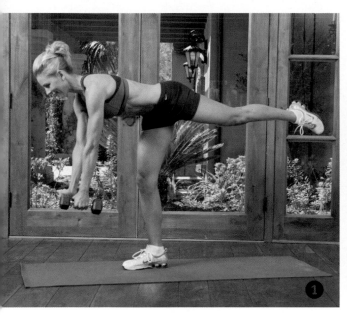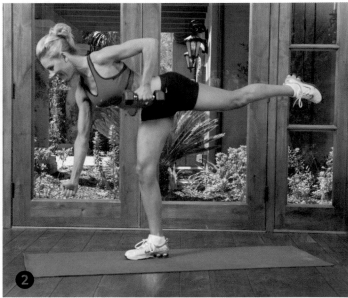

Benefits: Strengthens lats, rhomboids, legs, and core; improves balance

(1) Grab one medium-weight to heavy dumbbell and hold it in your left hand. Stand on your right leg and bring your left leg straight back and up so your torso and back leg are as parallel to the ground as you can get them. You may rotate the elevated foot internally for balance. Both arms should hang down toward the ground. This is your starting position.

(2) In this balancing position, pull the dumbbell straight up towards your back, squeeze your lats, and keep your core tight. Return to your starting position.

(3) Perform 12 to 15 repetitions on each leg and arm.

75 Single-Leg Dumbbell Reach (Intermediate/Advanced)

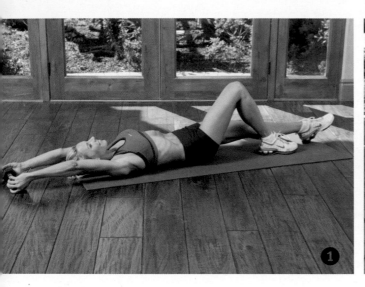 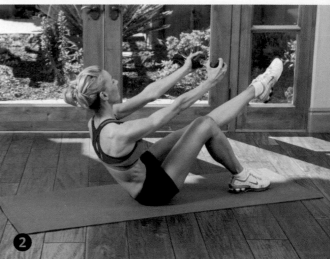

Benefits: Strengthens the rectus abdominis

① Lie on the floor with your right knee bent and your left leg extended on the floor. Hold one dumbbell between both hands over your head. This is your starting position.

② With your abdominals contracted, come up, raising and reaching the dumbbell toward your extended leg. At the same time, bring your extended leg up toward your dumbbell at the peak of the contraction. Return to your starting position.

③ Repeat the exercise for 12 to 15 repetitions, and then switch to the other leg.

Superman Flutters (Advanced)

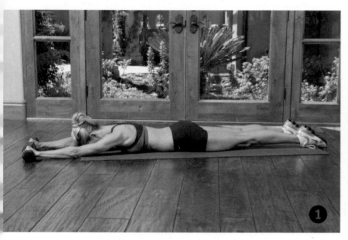

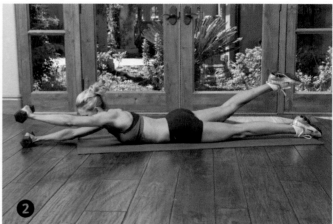

Benefits: Strengthens lower back, upper back, and glutes

(1) Lie facedown on the floor, holding light dumbbells in your hands with your arms extended straight overhead and your palms facing down. This is your starting position.

(2) Start the exercise by lifting opposite arms and legs off the floor at the same time, contracting your shoulder blades together, squeezing your glutes, and keeping your core tight. Your neck should stay neutral with a slight lift of your head. Repeat the fluttering until you have lifted each arm and leg for the same number of repetitions.

(3) Perform the exercise for 12 to 15 repetitions with each leg and arm.

77 Seated Bent-Over Single-Arm Rear Deltoid Raise (Beginner)

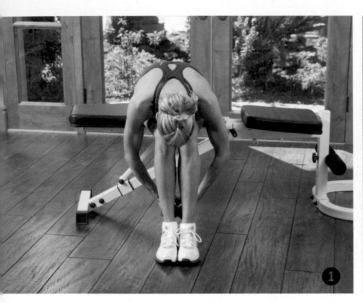 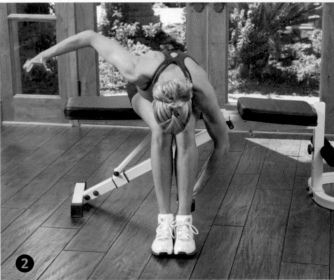

Benefits: Strengthens posterior deltoids

1. Sit on a bench with a dumbbell in one hand and bend over so your chest is resting on your thighs and your arms are down toward your shoes. This is your starting position.

2. Keeping your body stationary and your neck neutral, raise the dumbbell up and out laterally in an arching motion. Bring your arm back down and finish all repetitions on this arm before switching.

3. Complete 12 to 15 repetitions with each arm.

Plank Toe Taps (Advanced)

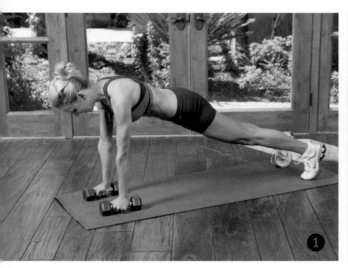 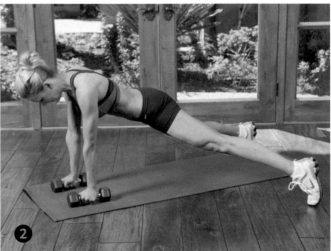

Benefits: Strengthens core, glutes, and legs

① Come to the floor in a plank position facing down, holding your dumbbells in your hands, arms straight, and wrists directly under your shoulders. You should be up on your toes as well. This is your starting position.

② While continuing to hold your plank position, begin by tapping your right toe out to the side and then right back to your center position.

③ Complete 15 to 20 repetitions with each leg.

79 Supine Bent-Knee Side-to-Side Rotation (All Levels)

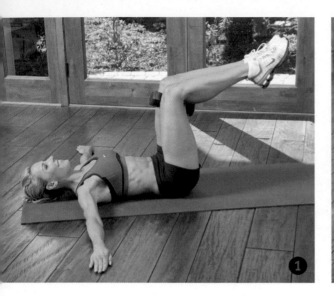 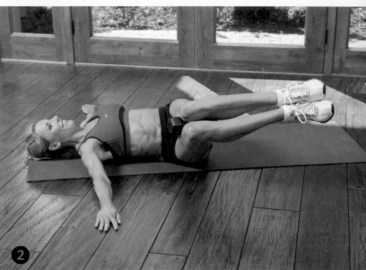

Benefits: Strengthens obliques, core, and hip flexors

① Grab one medium-weight dumbbell and come to the floor in a supine position, flat on your back, knees bent holding the dumbbell between them. Bring your legs up so they are in a 90-degree angle. Bring your arms out to your sides and rest them on the floor for balance. This is your starting position.

② While keeping the dumbbell tight between your knees, rotate from side to side, contracting your obliques as you go.

③ Complete the exercise by doing 15 to 20 repetitions on each side.

Plank Alternating Knee Tuck (Advanced)

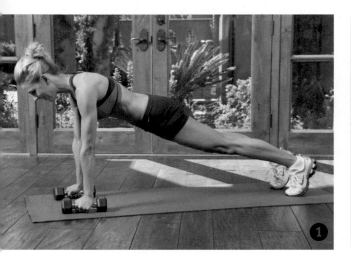

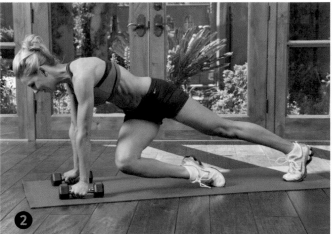

Benefits: Strengthens abdominals, obliques, and core

① Come to the floor in a plank position facing down, holding dumbbells in your hands, arms straight, and wrists directly under your shoulders. You should be up on your toes as well. This is your starting position.

② While maintaining a straight spine in plank position, bring one knee toward the opposite elbow. Extend the leg back to the starting position and then repeat this exercise on the opposite side.

③ Perform the exercise for 20 repetitions on each side.

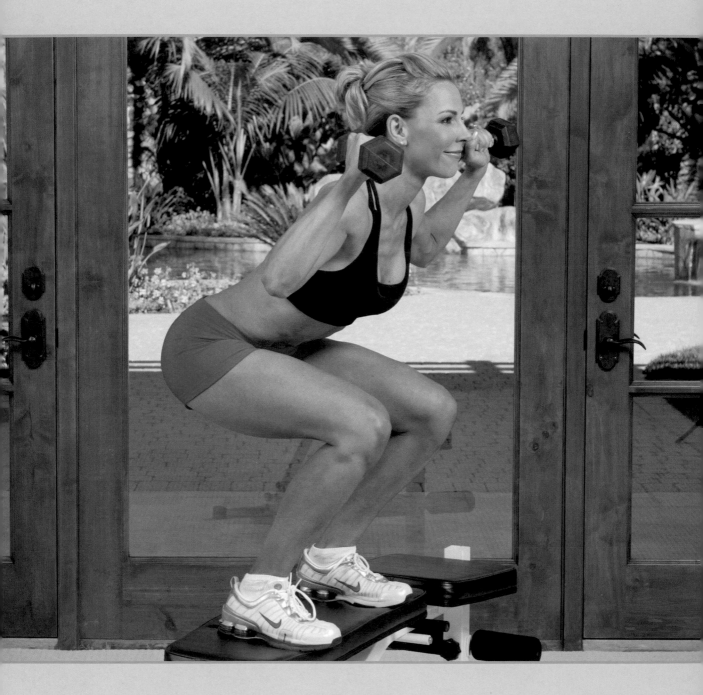

Compound Moves with Weights (Exercises 81–88)

CHAPTER 10

This is one of my favorite chapters because I am all about maximizing your time and efforts in your workouts! If you can, why not work more than one body part at a time, right? To make your body run more efficiently and become a fat-burning machine, you need to increase your metabolism. In order to speed this process up, we need to maximize our weight-lifting efforts. This is why these compound-move exercises are so great! If you have only five or ten minutes in the morning, don't fret! Any of these exercises would be a great way to start off your day right in a short amount of time.

Follow the same guidelines for choosing the correct amount of weight to use as outlined in chapters 5 and 6. Remember, when you get to the last three repetitions, you should be fatiguing the muscle. And remember what you learned about proper form in chapter 2. Keep your weight over the center of your body when appropriate for the exercise, stand tall with your shoulders back and down, pull in your rib cage rather than extending it, and pull your tummy in tight. It's important that you don't hyperextend your knee or elbow joints as this can increase potential injury to the joints.

When you are performing a compound move and working on a couple of muscles at once, I find that it's more difficult to concentrate on each individual muscle being worked. This is why it's very important to stay focused on the entire movement, from beginning to end. Practice the movement without any added weights, so you understand the directions in which you should be pushing or pulling (or both!). Concentrate on contracting your muscles at the peak of the movement. Make sure you never neglect the eccentric portion (when you are releasing the muscles and returning to your starting position), as your control on the latter half of the exercise is just as important as in the beginning. If you just throw your weights around without taking the time to understand the purpose and targeted muscles of the movement, you might as well not be working out at all!

And do I need to remind you to warm up? Go and visit chapter 4 again!

81 One-Two Punch with Lunge Kick (Advanced)

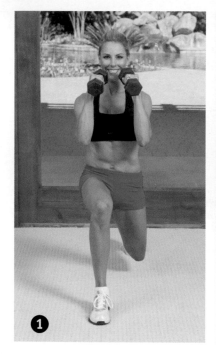
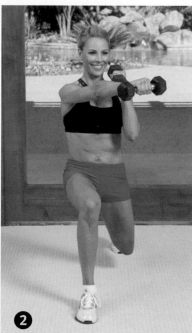
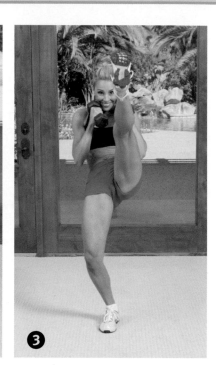

① **②** **③**

◎

Benefits: Strengthens quads, hamstrings, glutes, inner thighs, biceps, shoulders, and triceps

---

① Stand with a light dumbbell in each hand. Lunge forward with your right leg, bending your right knee 90 degrees and lowering your left knee to about 4 to 6 inches above the floor. Bring your dumbbells to chin level and keep your elbows down and palms in. This is your starting position.

② Punch your right hand diagonally, keeping your elbow slightly soft and turning your palm down; repeat with your left hand.

③ After the second punch, stand up, raising your left knee toward your chest, then kick forward with your left leg, pointing your toes. Lower back into a lunge and repeat.

④ Repeat the exercise for 12 to 15 repetitions with the same leg forward and then switch to the other leg and repeat.

Walking Lunge with Torso Rotation (Advanced)

82

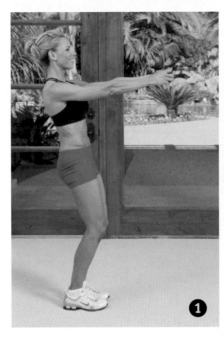 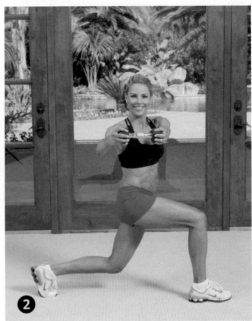

◎

Benefits: Strengthens glutes, quads, hamstrings, calves, core, and shoulders

---

① Begin by holding one medium-weight dumbbell in your hands. Lift the dumbbell straight up so your arms are parallel to the floor. This is your starting position. (Make sure you have room to perform 12 to 15 walking lunges forward before you begin.)

② Take one large step forward into a lunge position, with your knee at a 90-degree angle and the weight of your body in that front knee. Hold the lunge position, contract your abs, and rotate your torso to the same side as your forward leg. Your arms and dumbbell should turn with your torso until they are in line with your side. Rotate back to the center, and at the same time, stand back up and bring your arms back down in front of you.

③ Alternating sides, continue to do the walking lunges and rotations for 12 to 15 repetitions on each leg.

83 Plié and Calf Raise with Triceps Extensions (Beginner)

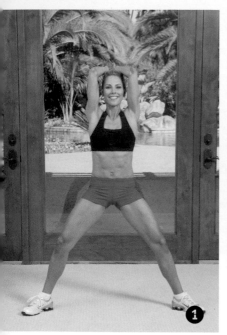
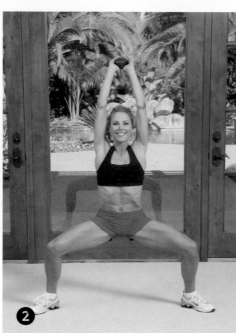
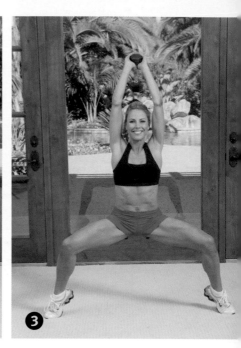

① ② ③

Benefits: Strengthens core, quads, hamstrings, outer and inner thighs, calves, lower back, and biceps

① Stand with one medium-weight to heavy dumbbell in your hands, lift it over your head with your elbows bent, and hang the dumbbell behind your head. Then bring your legs out wide with your toes and knees turned out. This is your starting position.

② Begin this exercise performing two moves at once. While extending your arms up and squeezing your triceps, bend down into a plié squat until your thighs are parallel to the floor. Keep your back tall and abs tight.

③ Hold this position and lift your heels off the ground, squeezing your calves. Pause for 2 seconds, put your heels back down, and lift up back to your starting position, including bringing your dumbbell back down behind your head.

④ Repeat this three-move exercise for 12 to 15 repetitions.

Alternating Lunges with a Row and Triceps Kickback Combo (Beginner)

84

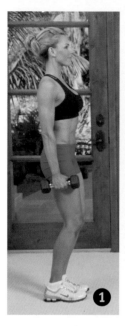 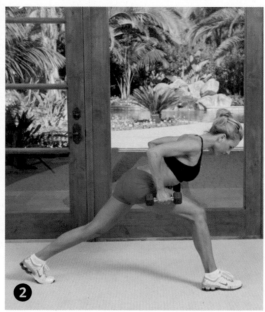 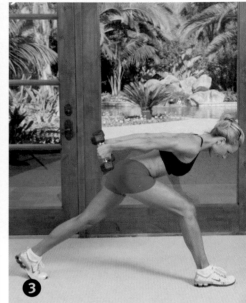

Benefits: Strengthens core, legs, upper back, and triceps

1. Stand holding a dumbbell in each hand down by your sides. This is your starting position.

2. Lunge forward with your right foot until your knee is at a 90-degree angle. Lean your body forward slightly and reach your arms and dumbbells down. First perform a row by lifting and bending your elbows towards your back, squeezing your back muscles.

3. Hold this position and begin your triceps kickback by holding your elbows in position and extending your arms back, squeezing your triceps.

4. Now reverse the entire exercise. Release your triceps kickback, extend your arms down, push off from your front heel and come back up to your standing position. Continue this entire exercise by alternating legs so you complete half of your repetitions on each leg. Try to complete 16 to 20 repetitions total.

85 Side Leg Lift and Lateral Shoulder Raise (Intermediate/Advanced)

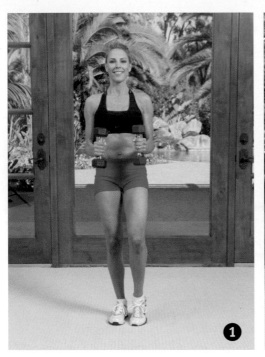 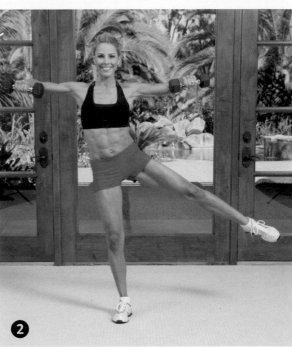

◎

Benefits: Strengthens core, outer thighs, hips, and shoulders

① Hold a dumbbell in each hand with your hands in front of your waist and your palms facing each other. Pull your shoulder blades back and put all your weight in your right foot. Raise the heel of your left foot so only the ball of your left foot is touching the floor. This is your starting position.

② Lift your left leg out laterally as high as you can without leaning, while at the same time lifting your arms out laterally, bringing your dumbbells up with your elbows slightly bent, but stopping when your forearms are parallel to the ground. Return to your starting position.

③ Repeat the exercise for 12 to 15 repetitions and then switch sides.

Step-Up with Squat and Shoulder Press (Advanced)

86

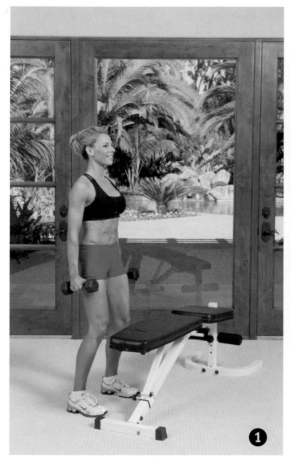
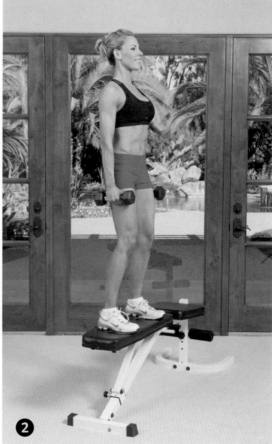

Benefits: Strengthens legs, shoulders, glutes, and core

(1) Grab two medium-weight to heavy dumbbells and hold them down at your sides. Stand at the side of a bench. This is your starting position.

(2) Begin by stepping up on top of the bench with your right leg. Make sure your heel comes all the way up so your entire foot is on top of the bench. Next bring your left foot up so both of your feet are stationary on top of the bench.

86 Step-Up with Squat and Shoulder Press (Advanced) continued

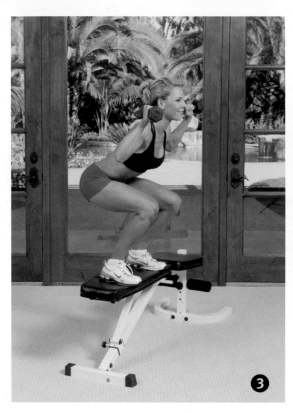

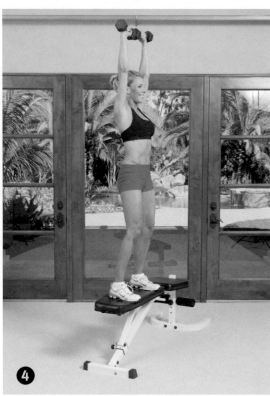

(3) Bring the dumbbells in front of your shoulders, palms facing forward. From this position, perform a squat by bending your knees and bringing your glutes down so your thighs are parallel to the ground and your knees are at a 90-degree angle.

(4) Push all the way up and at the same time perform an overhead shoulder press by pushing the dumbbells over your head. Bring the dumbbells back to your shoulders, step back down with the same leg that stepped up, and come back to your starting position.

(5) Repeat the entire exercise with the other leg leading. Alternate legs and complete the same number of repetitions on each side for 16 to 20 repetitions per side.

Squat Thrust Push-Up with Leg Lifts (Advanced)

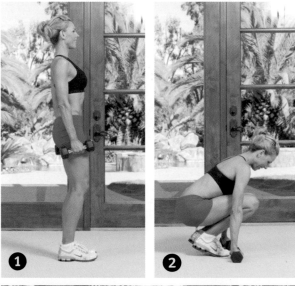

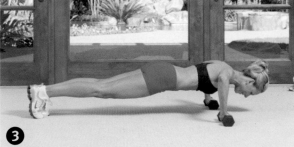

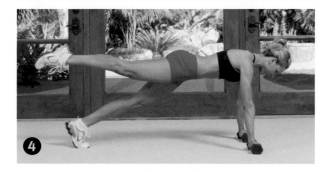

Benefits: Strengthens legs, glutes, core, and upper body

① Stand with your feet shoulder-width apart and your arms by your sides holding medium-weight dumbbells.

② Squat down, bringing your dumbbells to the floor outside your feet.

③ Jump your legs back into a plank pose and contract your abs. Do one push-up.

④ Hold at the top of the push-up position and lift one leg off the ground so that it is approximately parallel with the floor, squeezing your glute. Return your leg to the floor and switch legs, squeezing the other glute. Hop both feet back to the inside of your hands, and then jump up and push the dumbbells toward the ceiling in an overhead shoulder press.

⑤ Repeat the entire series for 12 to 15 repetitions.

88 Around the World Lunges with Biceps Curl (Advanced)

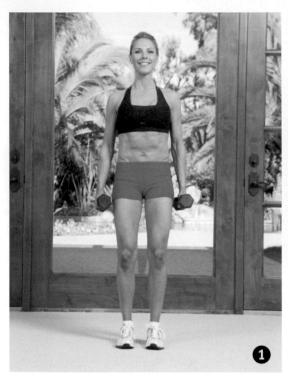

1

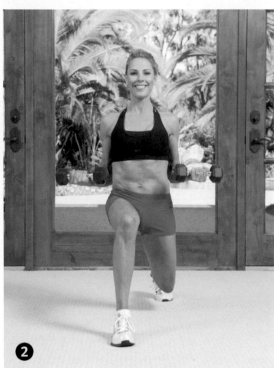

2

◎

Benefits: Strengthens legs, biceps, and core

① Begin by holding two medium-weight dumbbells in your hands with your arms extended down by your sides. This is your starting position. You will perform three different lunges while at the same time executing a biceps curl with each lunge by lifting your forearms to your shoulders and squeezing your biceps.

② The lunges will start with your right leg stepping forward and end with your knee at a 90-degree angle. At the same time, complete a biceps curl. Return to your starting position by pushing off your heel and returning your arms to their starting position.

88

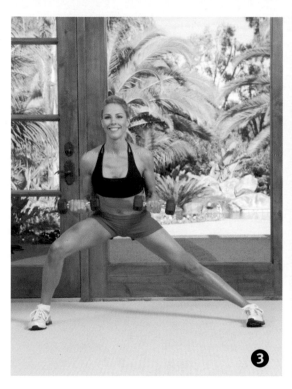

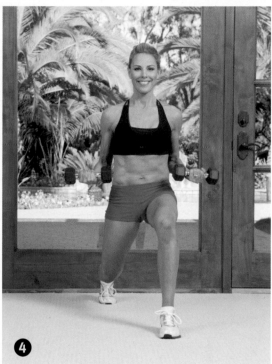

(3) The next lunge is a side lunge. Anchoring with your left leg and keeping it straight, your right leg lunges out to the side while you complete a biceps curl at the same time.

(4) The last lunge is a reverse lunge. Step your right leg straight back so your front leg is at a 90-degree angle. Again, complete a biceps curl with this lunge. Push back up with the heel of your left foot and return to your starting position.

(5) Complete all three lunges and biceps curls on one side, then switch sides. You should perform 12 to 15 repetitions on each side.

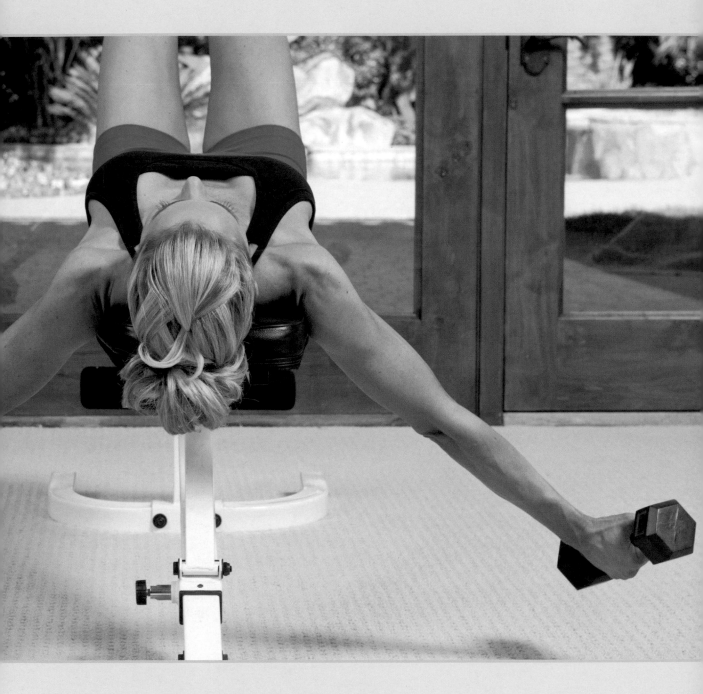

Weights with a Towel (Exercises 89–93)

I have been teaching fitness classes for more than sixteen years now. Sometimes doing the same exercises over and over can get a tad bit boring (for me as well as my students). This is why I try to think out-of-the-box and learn new moves from other classes or trainers. One of my Ultrafit personal trainers (thank you Dustin at Frog's Solana Beach!) used a towel during a class one day, and that got me thinking about how else it might be used. The reason the towel is so great is because if you use it on a slick surface, it makes for a sliding movement that requires control. This creates a whole new challenge for the exercise you do with it. Just like a stability ball, a towel requires you to use balance and your core as it creates a level of instability during an exercise to which your body must adapt. Like any other balancing exercises, being off-balance makes you engage many more muscles to keep from falling, giving you an amazing core workout without you even knowing it!

I came up with the following five exercises that incorporate not only dumbbells but a bath-size towel as well. I've included an upper-body exercise or abdominal exercise to go with each lower-body towel exercise to make the move even more intense. These exercises are definitely more advanced, so if you are a beginner, try some of the other workouts in the previous chapters to gain strength and control before jumping into the towel exercises.

For all of the exercises in this chapter, you will need a towel, a slick floor (wood, slate, tile, etc.), and medium to heavy weights. If you are having a difficult time with the towel exercises, try dropping down to lighter weights or take out the upper-body exercise that goes with it. Finally, don't forget to warm up! This should be fun—you've got to try at least one!

CHAPTER 11

89 Sliding Reverse Lunge and Shoulder Press (Beginner)

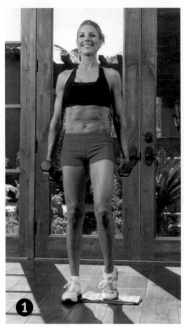
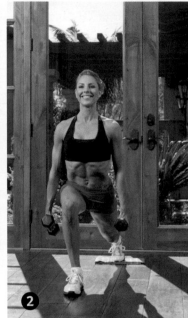
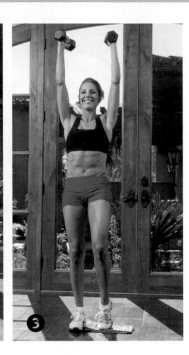

Benefits: Strengthens lower body, shoulders, and core

1. Begin by doubling up a towel, placing it on the floor, and putting your left toe on the towel. Your right foot will anchor next to your left toe and towel on the floor. Hold medium-weight to heavy dumbbells in your hands, down by your sides, and start by standing up tall. This is your starting position.

2. Start the exercise by sliding the towel by pushing your left leg back, keeping it straight, and stopping when your right leg is at a 90-degree angle. Return to your starting position and bend your arms so the dumbbells end at your shoulders with your elbows bent.

3. Keep your left knee slightly bent and lift both arms and dumbbells overhead, squeezing your shoulders, and then bring them back down to your sides.

4. Repeat the exercise for 12 to 15 repetitions on this side and then switch sides for the same amount of repetitions with the other leg.

Single-Leg Sliding Squat and Lateral Shoulder Raise (Beginner/Intermediate)

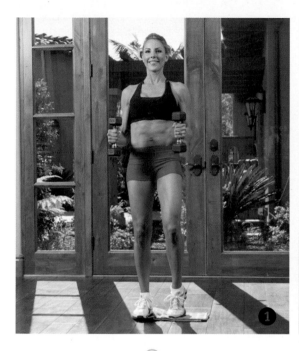 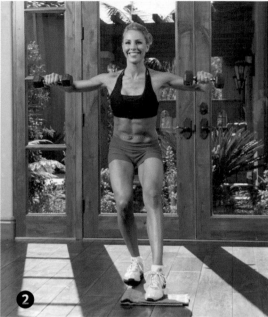

◎

Benefits: Strengthens legs, glutes, core, and shoulders

---

(1) Double up your towel and place it on the ground in front of you. Begin this exercise by holding two light to medium-weight dumbbells in your hands with your elbows bent, tucked into your sides, and arms at a 90-degree angle. Place your left foot on the towel, anchored with your right foot. This is your starting position.

(2) Start the exercise by sliding the towel with your left foot out in front of you by bending your right knee and performing a squat with that right leg. The weight of your body should remain in your right heel with your back as straight as you can make it. At the same time you do your sliding single-leg squat, lift your dumbbells out laterally, contracting your shoulders. Bring your arms back down and slide your left leg back in and stand back up.

(3) Repeat the exercise for 12 to 15 repetitions with your left leg on the towel and then complete the same number of reps with your right leg on the towel.

91 Sliding Side Lunge and Biceps Curl (Intermediate/Advanced)

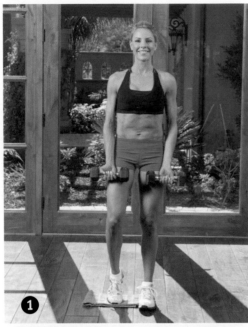

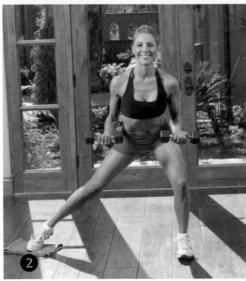

Benefits: Strengthens inner and outer thighs, glutes, legs, biceps, and core

① Begin by doubling up a towel and placing it on the floor under your right toe. Your left foot will anchor the move, and your weight should be placed in the heel of your left foot. Hold medium-weight to heavy dumbbells in your hands, with your arms extended down in front of your thighs and your palms facing forward. This is your starting position.

② Start the exercise by bending your left knee into a half squat and sliding the towel with your right foot out laterally to your right side, and performing biceps curls with both of your arms at the same time. Go as far out laterally as you can without compromising your form by dropping your shoulders or losing balance. The weight of your body should remain in your left heel, and your back should be as straight as you can make it. Now, contract your inner thigh and slide your right foot back in, while at the same time returning your arms down to their starting position (in front of your thighs) and standing back up.

③ Repeat the exercise for 12 to 15 repetitions with your right leg on the towel and then complete the same number of reps with your left leg.

Weighted Lower-Body Drag (Advanced)

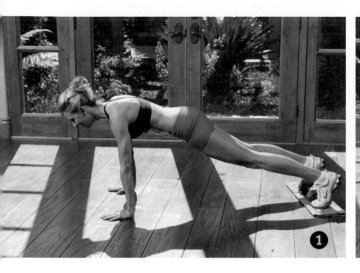

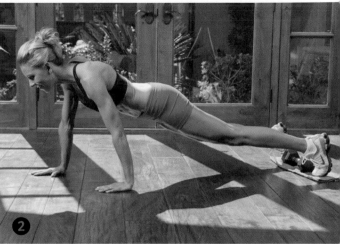

Benefits: Strengthens core, shoulders, legs, glutes, and upper body

(1) Begin this exercise by folding your towel in half and putting a medium-weight dumbbell in the center. Bring your body down with your hands on the floor and your feet on each side of the dumbbell and on the towel. Walk your hands out in front of you until your body is in a horizontal position, with your hands on the floor and your feet on the towel. This is your starting position.

(2) Before you begin, pull in your abs and pinch your shoulder blades behind. Maintain this strong core position throughout the exercise. Now walk your hands forward, pulling both the towel and dumbbell as you go.

(3) Walk your hands 12 to 15 steps forward.

Note: Make sure you have at least 20 feet of open space for this exercise.

93 Sliding Reverse Towel Ab Crunch (Advanced)

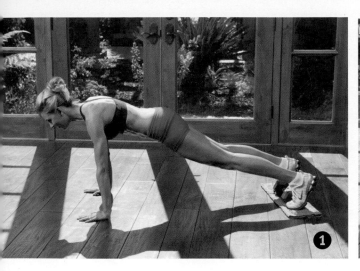
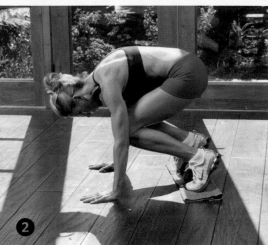

Benefits: Strengthens abs, core, upper body, legs

① Begin this core exercise by folding your towel in half and putting a medium-weight dumbbell in the center. Bring your body down with your hands on the floor and your feet on each side of the dumbbell and on the towel. Walk your hands out in front of you until your body is in a horizontal position, with your hands on the floor and your feet on the towel. This is your starting position.

② Before you begin, pull in your abs and pinch your shoulder blades behind. Maintain this strong core position throughout the exercise. Now keep your hands on the floor and pull your knees in to your chest, dragging the towel and dumbbell, exhale, hold for 1 second, and return to your starting position by sliding back the towel and dumbbell.

③ Repeat this exercise for 12 to 15 repetitions.

Weights for Yoga and Stretching (Exercises 94–101)

CHAPTER 12

In chapter 4, I discussed the importance of the preworkout warm-up, and the same ideas apply when you want to stretch. You always need to have warmed up for at least 5 to 10 minutes prior to stretching. Another option is to wait until the end of your workout to stretch. I prefer to stretch between sets as well as at the end of my workouts. That way, I'm improving my range of motion and helping to prevent injuries the entire time. Once you've gone through the motions of contracting your muscles in combination with weighted overload, you must stretch them to increase the length of the muscles and tendons to prevent injuries.

Yoga and stretching should be a big part of everyone's workout program. Not only do they help decrease muscle soreness and increase flexibility, but also it is a time to relax your mind and reflect on your day. When you lift weights or perform any of the workouts I have prepared for you in chapter 13, you might have some muscle soreness that is normal the day after lifting. Although weight-lifting injuries are rare, they sometimes happen. If you experience any of the following, take a few days off and see a medical professional if it doesn't resolve.

- Soreness that lasts more than two days and limits activity
- Pain worse on one side than the other
- Pain occurring in the joint, not in the muscle
- Swelling or bruising
- Loss of range of motion or mobility in the joint

The movements described below are some of my favorites. Using the dumbbells during the stretch allows me to get a deeper pull. Try them with the weights, but if you feel it might be too much, perform them without the weights and then add the weights back in when you have increased your strength and flexibility.

94

Supine Upper-Body Stretch on Bench (Beginner)

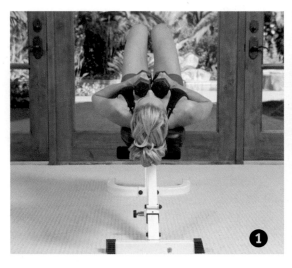

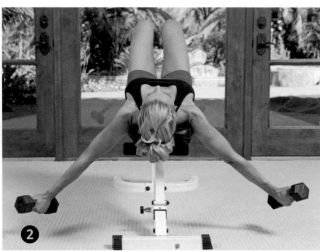

Benefits: Opens and stretches chest and upper back

① Hold two light to medium-weight dumbbells in your hands and lie down on a bench in a supine position with your head supported, your body in the center of the bench, and your feet planted on top of the bench. This is your starting position.

② Extend your arms up so that you're holding the dumbbells above your chest.

Inhale. On the exhale, lower your arms slowly until they are out to your sides and in a stretching position. Hold here, feeling your chest opening, your shoulders stretching, and your back releasing. Hold this position for 8 deep breaths, and then return to your starting position.

③ Repeat this stretch, each time stretching deeper, for 12 to 15 repetitions.

Seated Hip and Lower-Back Stretch (Beginner)

95

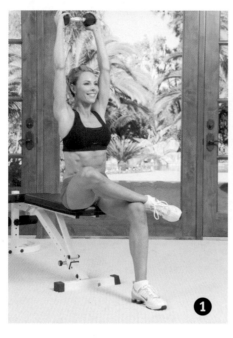
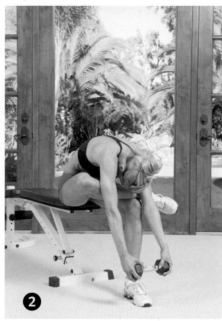

◎

Benefits: Stretches hips and back

---

① Hold one light to medium-weight dumbbell in both hands with your arms extended over your head. Sit on a bench with your right leg bent and your right ankle on your left knee and your left foot pressed firmly on the floor. This is your starting position.

② Begin by inhaling and bending your upper body slightly back, feeling a stretch in your shoulders and core muscles. Then exhale and bend from your hips, keeping your arms straight and bringing the dumbbell down in front of your right leg until you feel your lower back, right side hip, and hamstring stretch but not hurt. Hold this pose for 8 deep breaths and then return to the starting position.

③ Repeat for 12 to 15 repetitions with your right leg up and then switch for the same number of reps with your left leg up.

96

Standing Calf Stretch (Beginner)

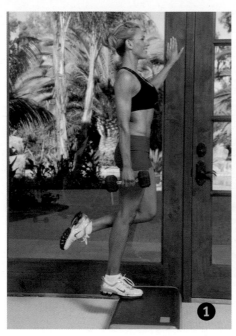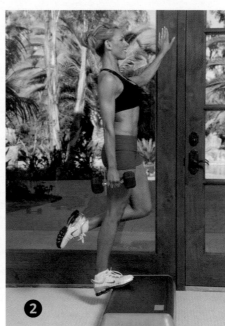

Benefits: Stretches calves and Achilles tendons

(1) Hold a medium-weight to heavy dumb-bell in your right hand and walk to a step or an elevated area where you can hold on to something for support. Hold on with your left hand, step onto the platform with both feet, and bring your right heel off the platform, with your knee slightly bent. Bend your left knee and lift your lower left leg up and back so only the right front half of your foot is on the platform. This is your starting position.

(2) Perform the single-leg calf stretch by inhaling and lifting your heel up, squeezing your calf muscle, and then returning to your starting position but allowing your heel to hang. Exhale and hold for 8 deep breaths.

(3) Repeat this movement for 12 to 15 rep-etitions on one leg and then switch sides. Each time, try to feel a deeper stretch.

Hanging Lower-Back/Hamstring Stretch (Intermediate)

97

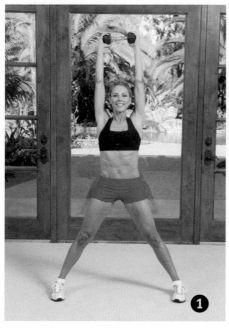

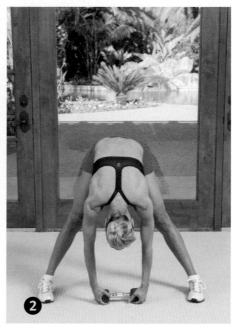

Benefits: Stretches lower back, hamstrings, shoulders, back, and neck

1. Hold one medium-weight dumbbell in both hands over your head and step your feet out wider than hip-width apart. Slightly turn your toes in and your heels out. This is your starting position.

2. Begin the stretch by leaning your entire body back, leading with the dumbbell over your head until you feel a stretch in your core. Pull your abs in and then exhale, and slowly perform a forward bend, keeping your arms straight and hips stationary until you are bent over and hanging the dumbbell down toward the ground. Relax your head, neck, and arms and remain there for 8 deep breaths and then slowly return to your starting position.

3. Repeat this exercise for 12 to 15 repetitions, trying to stretch deeper as you go.

98 Sliding Triangle Pose (Intermediate/Advanced)

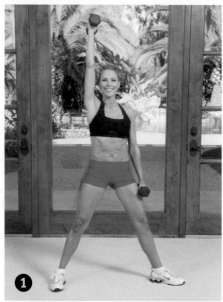

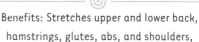

Benefits: Stretches upper and lower back, hamstrings, glutes, abs, and shoulders, and improves balance and core

1. Hold a light to medium-weight dumbbell in each hand and stand with your feet just wider than shoulder-width apart. Turn your left toes out to your left side, with your right toes pointing forward. Extend your left arm straight down, just outside your left thigh, and extend your right arm up straight overhead. Your legs should be straight but not totally locked out. This is your starting position.

2. Inhale, look up at your right arm, and shift your torso to the left. While exhaling, slowly slide your left arm and dumbbell down your left leg towards your shin or the floor (whatever your flexibility will allow), and then stop and hold that pose. Keep your right arm back in line with your body, but pull your top shoulder back to further stretch it and your abs. Hold the down position for 8 deep breaths. Keeping your eyes on the dumbbell in your right hand, slowly return to your starting position.

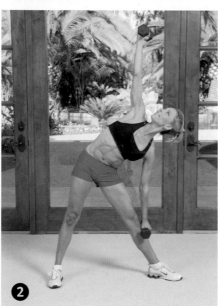

3. Repeat the exercise for 12 to 15 repetitions and then switch sides.

Extended Forward Lunge (Advanced)

99

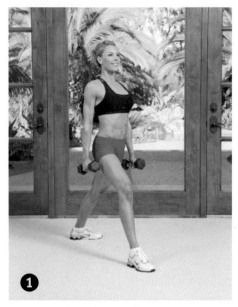

Benefits: Strengthens and tones thigh muscles, glutes, and upper body; stretches groin and leg muscles; and improves balance and core

1. Hold a light to medium-weight dumbbell in each hand, with your arms at your sides. Place your left foot behind you and your right leg in front. Turn your left foot out to your left side and keep your right foot facing forward. Try to make a straight line from your back leg to your front with your body in the center. This is your starting position.

2. From this position, inhale and then exhale into a front leg lunge so your knee is directly over your ankle and bent at a 90-degree angle. Square your hips forward, making sure your heels are aligned, and raise the dumbbells over your head with your palms facing each other, and look up at the dumbbells. Stretch tall and long into your hips and reach up nice and tall. Hold this position for 8 deep breaths and then return to your starting position.

3. Repeat for 12 to 15 repetitions on each leg.

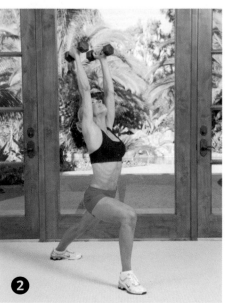

100 Extended Side Lunge and Reach (Intermediate/Advanced)

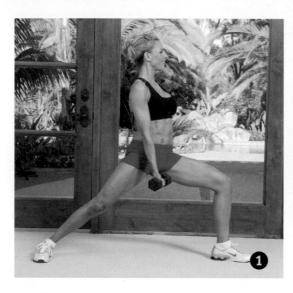 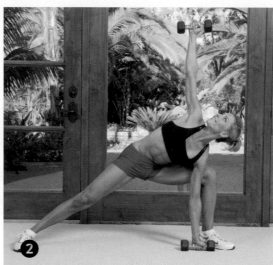

◎

Benefits: Strengthens and tones legs, thighs, ankles, and knees; stretches chest; and improves balance and core

(1) Hold a light to medium-weight dumbbell in each hand. Place your right foot behind you and your left leg in front. Turn your right foot out to your right side and keep your left foot facing forward. Try to make a straight line from your back leg to your front with your body in the center. From this position, inhale and then exhale into a front leg lunge so your knee is directly over your ankle and bent at a 90-degree angle. Square your hips forward, making sure

your heels are aligned. This is your starting position.

(2) From here, rotate your torso to the right, exhale, and allow your left dumbbell and arm to come to the floor, while at the same time your right arm and dumbbell will reach straight up. Your lunge might have to come lower, and you should look up at the right dumbbell on top. Hold this position for 8 deep breaths and then return to your starting position.

(3) Repeat this pose for 12 to 15 repetitions and then switch sides.

Alternating Bending Toe Reach (Intermediate/Advanced)

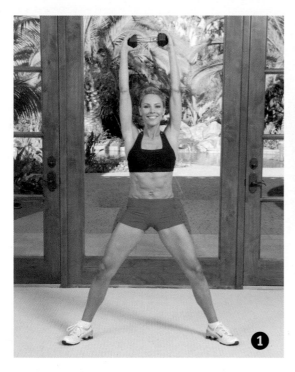

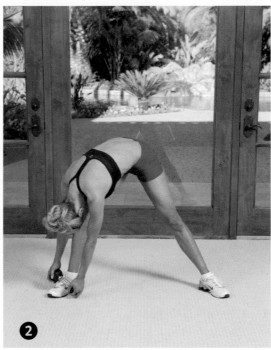

Benefits: Stretches shoulders

---

(1) Hold a light to medium-weight dumbbell in your hands over your head and step your feet out wider than hip-width apart. Keep your toes, feet, and knees turned slightly out. This is your starting Z position.

(2) Begin the stretch by inhaling, and then exhale and bend at your hips. With a circular-like motion, reach down with your arms and your dumbbell towards one foot and then hold. Relax and hold this position for 8 deep breaths, and then do a complete reverse motion back up to your starting position. Immediately perform the same move to the other foot and hold there for 8 deep breaths.

(3) Repeat this exercise, alternating sides, for 12 to 15 repetitions on each side.

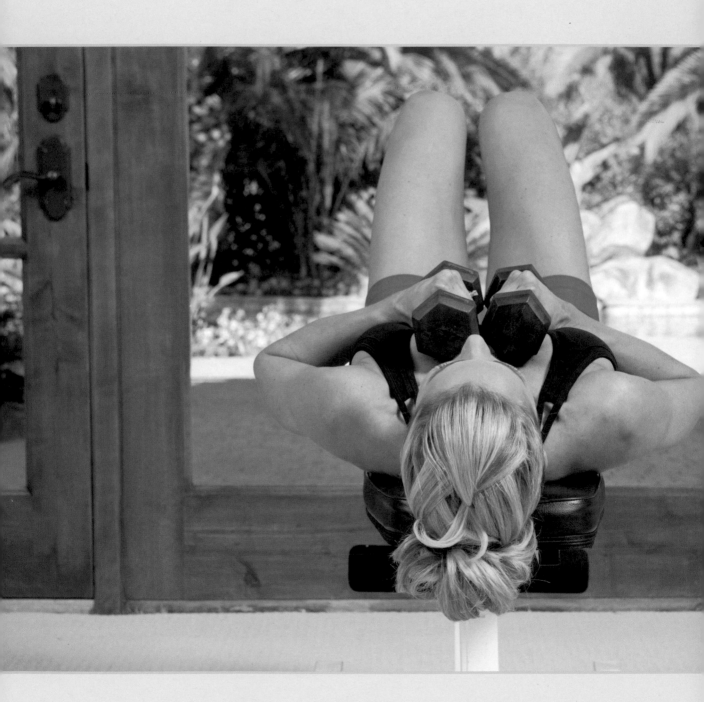

Creating Your Own Workouts

The secret to achieving the results you want is knowing how to combine exercises to create an effective total-body workout. The truly successful fitness professionals understand how to determine an individual's fitness level and create a program that suits his or her needs and abilities. We're always looking for maximum results! And from experience, I know that it's easy to become overwhelmed by the vast amount of information provided in a book like mine. I don't want you to give up, so I have created nineteen customized workouts using all 101 exercises in this book to make it easier for you to use them and maximize your time and efforts.

Now with that being said, I know most of my readers are more than capable of creating their own workouts using the 101 exercises I've provided. Go for it! Just make sure that when putting together your own workouts, you address the following questions:

1. What is my beginning level of fitness?

2. What are my short-term and long-term goals?

3. How much time do I realistically have for my workouts?

✳ Your Starting Fitness Level

There is something for everyone in this book. If you are a beginner, make sure you choose exercises classified as "beginner" or "all levels." You should be using lighter weights until your form and technique are properly developed. If you are at an intermediate or advanced level, make sure you're pushing yourself hard enough. Progressively increase your weights so that you're always exercising to fatigue. And make sure you use some of the more advanced exercises so that you see results and avoid a plateau.

✳ Setting Goals

I require all of my clients to determine baseline levels before beginning any fitness or nutrition program. This allows you to set realistic goals and develop a program that's both achievable and motivating. Anyone can look in a mirror and be dissatisfied with one body part or another, but it's much more important to look at the whole picture.

✳ Time Management

Mapping your workout plan onto a month-long calendar can be very useful because it helps you to visualize the overall time commitment you'll need to make. From there, I suggest writing down your fitness plan every Sunday for the week to come. This allows you to reorganize your schedule (if it's like mine, it's *always* changing), look at your calendar, and see what your week is going to be like. In addition, I suggest that you maintain a workout log, which allows you to check in on your progress toward meeting your goals and see what you're doing right or wrong.

Always block out time within each day for a scheduled workout. Now, did you notice I said *every day*? Even if you are crazy busy, you can find 5 minutes within your day to do something! Try the 5-Minute Abs Workout or the 5-Minute Arms and Abs Workout on those busy days. Inevitably, you're going to have a day where you can't fit anything else in, you're too tired, or your child is sick, etc. This will end up being your rest day. Obviously, if you get to the end of your week and nothing has prevented you from fitting in your workouts, you'll need to take a rest day over the weekend. And please, if you know that you tend to be too tired in the evenings, or you can't get out of bed in the mornings, *don't* schedule your workout for then unless you absolutely have to! Your workouts may not always feel good, but they are your time to relax and release and settle your mind and body for either the day ahead, or from the day you just left behind. Enjoy this time! When you feel better about yourself, your whole day will go better!

Once you acknowledge your starting points, you can then determine the workouts you need to use in order to meet your goals, as well as how much time you have to devote to your training. Review the body type descriptions I provided in chapter 3 so that you can correctly utilize the body type–specific workouts I've provided in this chapter. There are a multitude of options available to you within this book to help you reach your goals!

✳ The Workouts

WORKOUT 1: 5-Minute Abs (All Levels)

#71 Half sit-up

#78 Plank toe taps

#79 Supine bent-knee side-to-side rotation

WORKOUT 2: 5-Minute Arms and Abs (All Levels)

#11 Dumbbell push-up

#20 Seated incline crunch and biceps curl

#26 Balancing single-leg triceps kickback

WORKOUT 3: 10-Minute Glutes (All Levels)

#38 Pulsing diagonal reverse lunge and lift

#37 Elevated lunge

#36 Donkey glute kick

#32 Bridge and scoop

#95 Seated hip and lower-back stretch

WORKOUT 4: 10-Minute Total-Body Fat Blaster (Intermediate)

#11 Dumbbell push-up

#5 Alternating front lunge and torso twist

#66 Squat and jump shoulder press

#81 One-two punch with lunge kick

#22 Balancing single-leg alternating biceps curl

WORKOUT 5: 10-Minute Power Stretch (All Levels)

#3 Wood chop

#98 Sliding triangle pose

#99 Extended forward lunge

#100 Extended side lunge and reach

#101 Alternating bending toe reach

WORKOUT 6: 15-Minute Ab Blast (Intermediate/Advanced)

#1 Torso twist

#68 Frontal plane oblique side bend

#80 Plank alternating knee tuck

#73 Side oblique dumbbell rotation

#54 Supine gator rotation

#55 Long-lever trunk curl

WORKOUT 7: 15-Minute Leg Toner (All Levels)

#30 Single-leg step-up

#29 Single-leg bullet squat

#31 Prone hamstring curl

#43 Multi-rep seated calf raise

#27 Modified sissy squat

#41 Side-plank triangle lift

WORKOUT 8: 15-Minute Upper-Body Strengthener (All Levels)

#2 Alternating front punch

#8 Dumbbell pullover

#12 Multi-repetition incline chest press

#15 Dumbbell upright row into alternating single-arm press

#19 Seated single-arm concentration curl

#23 Skull crushers

WORKOUT 9: 15-Minute Butt Blaster (Intermediate/Advanced)

#63 Plié pop-up

#35 Reverse lunge torso twist

#34 Single-leg dead lift

#59 Reverse rolling single-leg lunge

#58 Hip raise

#99 Extended forward lunge

WORKOUT 10: 15-Minute Posture/Core Strengthener (All Levels)

#70 Alternating bent-over row with supinated wrists

#77 Seated bent-over single-arm rear deltoid raise

#17 Balancing single-leg rear delt fly

#76 Superman flutters

#72 Prone rear deltoid raise

#46 Hyperextension

#49 Stability ball cobra

#57 Oblique cross chop

WORKOUT 11: 30-Minute Total Body Toner (Intermediate/Advanced)

#4 Squat into overhead shoulder press

#10 Straight-arm pullover with one leg out

#14 Dumbbell fly with supinated wrists

#21 Side-lunge single-arm concentration curl

#83 Plié and calf raise with triceps extensions

#87 Squat thrust push-up with leg lifts

#75 Single-leg dumbbell reach

#80 Plank alternating knee tuck

#97 Hanging lower-back/hamstring stretch

#100 Extended side lunge and reach

WORKOUT 12: 30-Minute Upper-Body Toner (All Levels)

#1 Torso twist

#45 Stability ball upper-back pump

#9 One-arm row from plank position

#7 Incline bench row

#47 Supine bridge chest press

#50 Alternating overhead extensions, one leg up

#52 Stability ball preacher curl

#25 Supine bridge single-leg triceps extension

#18 Side-lying, internal-rotation rear deltoid raise

#94 Supine upper-body stretch on bench

WORKOUT 13: 30-Minute Lower-Body Blast (All Levels)

#3 Wood chop

#82 Walking lunge with torso rotation

#65 Single-arm power clean

#28 Seated leg extension

#33 Single-arm cross dead lift

#42 Alternating front curtsy lunge

#43 Multi-rep seated calf raise

#39 Side-lying inner-thigh lift

#97 Hanging lower-back/hamstring stretch

#96 Standing calf stretch

WORKOUT 14:
30-Minute Interval Calorie Burner (Intermediate/Advanced)

#6 Alternating side lunge and shoulder press

#62 Dumbbell run

#64 Lateral shuffling dumbbell switch

#63 Plié pop-up

#48 Alternating chest fly, one leg up

#84 Alternating lunges with a row and triceps kickback combo

#85 Side leg lift and lateral shoulder raise

#86 Step-up with squat and shoulder press

#88 Around the world lunges with biceps curl

#61 Toe calf running

#99 Extended forward lunge

WORKOUT 15: 30-Minute Glutes and Abs (Intermediate/Advanced)

#5 Alternating front lunge and torso twist

#37 Elevated lunge

#56 Crunch with rotation

#58 Hip raise

#60 Forward sliding single-leg squat

#78 Plank toe taps

#32 Bridge and scoop

#67 Frog-legs ab crunch

#98 Sliding triangle pose

#95 Seated hip and lower-back stretch

WORKOUT 16: 30-Minute Ectomorph Workout (All Levels)

#28 Seated leg extension

#31 Prone hamstring curl

#66 Squat and jump shoulder press

#44 Single-leg elevated heel raise

#20 Seated incline crunch and biceps curl

#12 Multi-repetition incline chest press

#24 Bent-over double-arm triceps kickback

#69 Bent-over rear delt into back rows

#75 Single-leg dumbbell reach

#100 Extended side lunge and reach

WORKOUT 17: 30-Minute Endomorph Workout (All Levels)

#2 Alternating front punch

#16 Shoulder 3-phase move

#10 Straight-arm pullover with one leg out

#77 Seated bent-over single-arm rear deltoid raise

#74 Balancing single-leg bent-over row

#83 Plié and calf raise with triceps extensions

#34 Single-leg dead lift

#35 Reverse lunge torso twist

#36 Donkey glute kick

#54 Supine gator rotation

#97 Hanging lower-back/hamstring stretch

WORKOUT 18: 30-Minute Mesomorph Workout (All Levels)

#62 Dumbbell run

#64 Lateral shuffling dumbbell switch

#87 Squat thrust push-up with leg lifts

#53 Elevated triceps dips

#80 Plank alternating knee tuck

#40 Supine bridge leg extension

#55 Long-lever trunk curl

#98 Sliding triangle pose

#99 Extended forward lunge

#100 Extended side lunge and reach

#101 Alternating bending toe reach

WORKOUT 19: Bonus: Creative Towel Combo (Intermediate/Advanced)

#89 Sliding reverse lunge and shoulder press

#90 Single-leg sliding squat and lateral shoulder raise

#91 Sliding side lunge and biceps curl

#92 Weighted lower-body drag

#93 Sliding reverse towel ab crunch

Nutrition

Let me begin this chapter by saying that if you only exercise and don't adhere to a good nutrition program, you're doing yourself a disservice. In all my years of personal training and nutritional consulting, as well as training my own body, I've always said that diet is 70 percent of how your body looks and feels. It's proven to me time and time again as I see the same people in the gym working out every day, sometimes for hours at a time, and never showing any visible results in their body composition.

Ultimately, any weight-loss effort requires that you create a caloric deficit, either through increased exercise or decreased caloric intake, or preferably a combination of the two. The best combination is a moderate caloric reduction and a larger increase of activity. In order to succeed, you need to keep your metabolism from slowing down. To do that, you must keep eating! The key is to eat the right foods, such as lean proteins, complex carbohydrates, and essential fats, and to make sure you're eating often enough (five or six smaller meals). Additionally, exercise increases your caloric expenditure and helps speed that metabolism up.

But you may not know how many calories you should be taking in each day. Your very first step should be to keep a food log for at least three days, if not a week. This will allow you to really embrace how much you're eating on a daily basis (and how much more or less you *should* be eating!). Nothing is more important than listening to your body's needs and using common sense to determine appropriate caloric intake levels, especially as workouts grow in both intensity and duration. You *must* be willing to be flexible, and at set points in your program (e.g., three weeks, six weeks, etc.), it's extremely important that you take the time to recalculate your BMI (body mass index) and make sure you're on the correct path toward your goals.

✳ Calculating Body Composition and Caloric Intake

Body composition refers to the relative amount of muscle, fat, bone, and other vital parts of the body. A scale by itself can be extremely misleading (since muscle weighs more than fat). It's far more important to look at changing your body from many different angles, and to provide yourself with starting points from which to determine your progress. As a result, you'll be able to set goals and determine when you've reached them!

Step #1: Body Mass Index (BMI)*

The following mathematical formula provides a measure of body fat based on both height and weight, and it applies to both men and women. BMI equals a person's weight in kilograms, divided by a person's height in meters squared: BMI = Weight (kg)/Height (m2). However, BMI uses total body weight instead of estimating fat and lean body mass separately, so it does not discriminate between individuals who have excess adipose tissue (overfat) and individuals with more athletic and muscular body types. Keep this in mind! This is only *one* form of body composition measurement!

You can do the math yourself, or you can use the table on page 169, which has already done the math and metric conversions. To use the table, find your height in the left-hand column. Move across the row to your weight. The number at the top of the column is the BMI for your height and weight.

***VERY IMPORTANT REMINDER:** Since BMI uses total body weight instead of estimating fat and lean body mass separately, it does not discriminate between individuals who have excess adipose tissue (overfat) and individuals with more athletic and muscular body types.

BMI (kg/m2)	19	20	21	22	23	24	25	26	27	28	29	30	35	40
Height (in.)							Weight (lb.)							
58	91	96	100	105	110	115	119	124	129	134	138	143	167	191
59	94	99	104	109	114	119	124	128	133	138	143	148	173	198
60	97	102	107	112	118	123	128	133	138	143	148	153	179	204
61	100	106	111	116	122	127	132	137	143	148	153	158	185	211
62	104	109	115	120	126	131	136	142	147	153	158	164	191	218
63	107	113	118	124	130	135	141	146	152	158	163	169	197	225
64	110	116	122	128	134	140	145	151	157	163	169	174	204	232
65	114	120	126	132	138	144	150	156	162	168	174	180	210	240
66	118	124	130	136	142	148	155	161	167	173	179	186	216	247
67	121	127	134	140	146	153	159	166	172	178	185	191	223	255
68	125	131	138	144	151	158	164	171	177	184	190	197	230	262
69	128	135	142	149	155	162	169	176	182	189	196	203	236	270
70	132	139	146	153	160	167	174	181	188	195	202	207	243	278
71	136	143	150	157	165	172	179	186	193	200	208	215	250	286
72	140	147	154	162	169	177	184	191	199	206	213	221	258	294
73	144	151	159	166	174	182	189	197	204	212	219	227	265	302
74	148	155	163	171	179	186	194	202	210	218	225	233	272	311
75	152	160	168	176	184	192	200	208	216	224	232	240	279	319
76	156	164	172	180	189	197	205	213	221	230	238	246	287	328

BMI Present Date:	BMI Halfway to Goal Date:	BMI at Goal Date:

After determining your BMI, check out the classification categories on the chart below. If you are a beginner and have a BMI greater than 29.9, I encourage you to get approval from your personal physician prior to starting any of the exercise programs in this book.

BMI Classifications and Risk of Associated Disease according to BMI and Waist Size

Classification	BMI (kg/m2)	Obesity Class	Disease Risk	Waist Less Than or Equal to 40 in. (men) 35 in. (women)	Waist Greater Than 40 in. (men) or or 35 in. (women)
Underweight	<18.5		Increased	-----	-----
Healthy Weight	18.5–24.9		-----	-----	-----
Overweight	25–29.9		Increased	Increased	High
Obesity	30–34.9 35–39.9	I II	High Very High	Very High Very High	High Very High
Extreme Obesity	>40	III	Extremely High	Extremely High	Extremely High

Step #2: Circumference Measures

Using a nonelastic measuring tape, record your measurements below:

Measurement Location	Inches Present Date:	Inches Halfway to Goal Date:	Inches at Goal Date:
Shoulders			
Chest			
Bicep			
Forearm			
Waist			
Hips			
Upper Thigh			
Lower Thigh			
Calf			

Step #3: Before/After Photos

Measurements provide you with numbers to keep track of, but photos speak the truth. You'll have the pleasure of seeing the results of all of your hard workouts with before and after photos. Gather your courage, put on your smallest bathing suit, and take some photos.

Step #4: Body Fat Calculator

Visit www.ultrafitnutrition.com to use our online body fat calculator.

Body Fat Present Date:	Body Fat Halfway to Goal Date:	Body Fat at Goal Date:

✳ Daily Guidelines to Follow for Success

Daily "Dos"

- DO drink more water. The range, depending upon the individual and daily level of activity, should be between 60 and 128 ounces of water per day.

- DO take an essential oil (Ultra-Omega Oil) along with water-soluble nutrients (Ultra-Power Packs) that together complete your fat-soluble and water-soluble nutrient needs every day.

- DO eat breakfast—*no skipping meals!*

- DO try to limit the amount of fruit you eat to one or two pieces per day, and always add in both a protein and fat source.

- DO eat two complex carbohydrates per day, preferably at breakfast and lunch, and make sure to combine them with both a protein and fat source.

- DO eat every three hours, five or six times a day, and try not to snack in between.

- DO choose a lean protein source, such as chicken, fish, or turkey, at every meal.

- DO go for food that is grilled, poached, baked, or steamed.

- DO get sauce on the side so you have control over your portions.

- DO drink two glasses of water before your meal when eating out, and always order a salad with low-fat or nonfat dressing on the side.

- DO say no to cheese, butter, or any type of white sauce when eating out.

- DO plan what you're going to eat and what you need to bring with you the night before so as to avoid making poor food choices due to lack of planning.

- DO take bottled water, apples, almonds, low-sugar protein bars, and any of your supplements in the car and whenever you travel away from home.

Daily "Don'ts"

- DON'T break away from eating nonfat or low-fat dairy products.

- DON'T go near white sauces, egg yolks, processed foods, white flour, white rice, or potatoes when you're following this plan.

- DON'T consume simple sugars or high-sugar fruits such as raisins and bananas when you're following this plan.

- DON'T overdo it on salad dressing—two to three tablespoons of low-fat or nonfat dressing is all you need!

- DON'T eat two to three hours before going to bed if you can help it.

- DON'T drink more than one beverage with caffeine a day.

- DON'T eat more than one protein bar a day, and try to keep it to half a bar at a sitting.

- DON'T consume more than twenty to thirty grams of fat per day, and limit your saturated fat intake to 10 percent of your total daily intake.

- DON'T let yourself get dehydrated—it can cause irritability, fatigue, false hunger, headaches, and much more!

✳ Ultrafit Quick-Start Weight-Loss Menu

The Quick-Start menu was designed as a great way to begin your diet, but was noot intended to be a maintenance program. Due to the low-calorie intake of this menu it is most appropriate for women. Men should add anywhere between 400-600 calories to this diet to insure adequate nutrition.

Ultrafit Sample Menu Plan: Day 1

Quantity	Description	Calories
Breakfast		
1 slice	Bread, whole wheat	120.00
3	Egg whites, scrambled/boiled	51.00
1 Tbsp	Essential Oil and Nutrients	120.00
1 Tbsp	Jelly, low sugar	25.00
		316.00
AM Snack		
15	Almonds	104.04
1	Apple, medium with peel	81.00
		185.04
Lunch		
1.5 cups, diced or chopped	Broccoli	36.96
0.5 cup	Brown rice, cooked	110.00
0.75 cup	Tuna, solid white in water	210.00
		356.96

PM Snack		
0.5 cup	Blueberries	40.60
0.5 cup	Nonfat cottage cheese	80.00
1 cup	Green tea	0.00
		120.60
Dinner		
1 cup	Salad (any veggies)	49.00
2 Tbsp	Reduced-calorie dressing	40.00
6 ounces	Ultrafit Nutrition Systems Barbecue Roasted Salmon (recipe to follow)	314.00
		403.00
		TOTAL: 1,381.60

Everyday, take:

- Essential oil*

- Nutrients

- 60 to 128 ounces water

- Green tea with afternoon snacks

*My clients take Ultra Essential Oil. It's important for regulating blood sugar; improving digestion; controlling sugar cravings; strengthening and lubricating ligaments, tendons, and joints; maintaining a healthy hormonal balance; and healing and preventing stretch marks and skin problems. Ultra Essential Oil contains rice, soy, sunflower, pumpkin, wheat germ, and olive oils, and it can be bought in the products section of www.ultrafitnutrition.com.

Day 1 Recipes

Ultrafit Nutrition Systems Barbecue Roasted Salmon

$\frac{1}{2}$ cup (60 ml) pineapple juice

2 tablespoons (30 ml) fresh lemon juice

4 (6-ounce, or 170-g) salmon fillets

2 tablespoons (25 g) brown sugar

4 teaspoons chili powder

2 teaspoons grated lemon rind

$\frac{1}{2}$ teaspoon ground cumin

$\frac{1}{2}$ teaspoon salt

$\frac{1}{2}$ teaspoon ground cinnamon

Cooking spray

Lemon slices (optional)

1. Combine the pineapple juice, lemon juice, and salmon in a zip-top plastic bag; seal and marinate in the refrigerator for 1 hour, turning occasionally.

2. Preheat the oven to 400°F (200°C, or gas mark 6).

3. Remove fish from bag; discard marinade. Combine the brown sugar, chili powder, lemon rind, cumin, salt, and cinnamon in a bowl. Rub over fish; place in an 11 x 7-inch (28 x 17¹/2-cm) baking dish coated with cooking spray. Bake for 12 minutes or until fish flakes easily when tested with a fork. Serve with lemon slices, if desired.

Serving size: 6-ounce (170-g) fillet, calories: 314, protein: 35.30 grams, carbs: 9 grams, fat: 14.7 grams

Ultrafit Sample Menu Plan: Day 2

Quantity	Description	Calories
Breakfast		
1 Tbsp	Essential Oil and Nutrients	120.00
0.5 scoop	Vanilla Protein Powder	55.00
0.5 cup	Milk, nonfat	40.00
0.5 cup	Oatmeal, quick, measured uncooked	140.00
		355.00
AM Snack		
15	Almonds	104.04
1	Plum, fresh, 2.25" diameter	36.00
		140.04
Lunch		
4 ounces	Chicken breast (white meat)	187.00
1 large (3 ¹/2" long, 3" diameter)	Pepper, sweet, yellow, raw	50.22
1 cup	Yam, baked or broiled	158.00
		395.22
PM Snack		
1 cubic inch	Cheese, low-fat, Cheddar or Colby	29.41
4	Melba toasts, wheat, unsalted	66.67
2 ounces	Turkey breast (white meat)	76.50
1 cup	Green tea	0.00
		172.58

Quantity	Description	Calories
Dinner		
1 ½ cups	Chicken Tortilla Soup	310.28
		1310.28
		TOTAL: 1,373.12

Everyday, take:

- Essential oil*
- Nutrients
- 60 to 128 ounces water
- Green tea with afternoon snacks

*My clients take Ultra Essential Oil. It's important for regulating blood sugar; improving digestion; controlling sugar cravings; strengthening and lubricating ligaments, tendons, and joints; maintaining a healthy hormonal balance; and healing and preventing stretch marks and skin problems. Ultra Essential Oil contains rice, soy, sunflower, pumpkin, wheat germ, and olive oils, and it can be bought in the products section of www.ultrafitnutrition.com.

Ultrafit Sample Menu Plan: Day 3

Quantity	Description	Calories
Breakfast		
1 cubic inch	Cheese, low-fat, Cheddar or Colby	29.41
1 ½ cups	Milk, nonfat	51.00
1 Tbsp	Essential Oil and Nutrients	120.00
0.5 cup	Salsa, ready to serve	18.20
1	Tortilla, corn, soft, 7" diameter	45.00
		263.61
AM Snack		
1 scoop	Whey Vanilla Protein Powder	110.00
1 cup	Milk, nonfat	80.00
1 cup	Strawberries	60.00
	Ice to blend in blender	250.00
Lunch		
1 ½ cups	Chicken Tortilla Soup	310.28
		310.28

PM Snack		
15	Almonds	104.04
0.5 Tbsp	Cinnamon, ground	8.87
0.5 cup	Oatmeal, quick, measured uncooked	140.00
		252.91
Dinner		
1 cup	Asparagus, raw	30.82
1 Cup	Ultrafit Nutrition Systems Broiled Sea Bass with Pineapple Chili-Basil Glaze (recipe to follow)	208.00
		238.82
1	Low-sugar Fudgsicle	45.00
		45.00
		TOTAL: 1,360.62

Everyday, take:

- Essential oil*

- Nutrients

- 60 to 128 ounces water

- Green tea with afternoon snacks

*My clients take Ultra Essential Oil. It's important for regulating blood sugar; improving digestion; controlling sugar cravings; strengthening and lubricating ligaments, tendons, and joints; maintaining a healthy hormonal balance; and healing and preventing stretch marks and skin problems. Ultra Essential Oil contains rice, soy, sunflower, pumpkin, wheat germ, and olive oils, and it can be bought in the products section of www.ultrafitnutrition.com.

Day 3 Recipes

Ultrafit Nutrition Systems Broiled Sea Bass with Pineapple Chili-Basil Glaze

3 tablespoons (60 g) pineapple preserves

2 tablespoons (30 ml) rice vinegar

1 teaspoon chopped fresh or 1/2 teaspoon dried basil

1/8 teaspoon crushed red pepper

1 garlic clove, minced

1/2 teaspoon salt, divided

4 (6-ounce, or 170-g) sea bass or other firm white fish fillets (about 1-inch, or 2.5 cm, thick)

1/2 teaspoon black pepper

Cooking spray

1. Preheat broiler.

2. Combine the preserves, vinegar, basil, red pepper, garlic, and ½ teaspoon of the salt in a small bowl.

3. Sprinkle the fillets with the remaining ½ teaspoon of salt and the black pepper. Place the fillets on a broiler pan coated with cooking spray; broil for 5 minutes. Remove from oven; brush fillets evenly with glaze. Return to oven; broil for an additional 5 minutes, or until the fish flakes easily when tested with a fork.

Serving size: 6-ounce (170-g) fillet, calories: 208, protein: 31.40 grams, carbs: 10.70 grams, fat: 3.4 grams

Ultrafit Sample Menu Plan: Day 4

Quantity	Description	Calories
Breakfast		
0.5	Bagel, wheat	60.00
3	Egg whites, scrambled/boiled	51.00
1 Tbsp	Cream cheese, nonfat	10.00
1 Tbsp	Essential Oil and Nutrients	120.00
		241.00
AM Snack		
1	Grapefruit, pink or red, 4" diameter	92.00
0.5	Low-sugar protein bar (I like Trioplex bars and The Doctor's Diet Carb Rite bars)	168.00
		260.00
Lunch		
1 cubic inch	Cheese, feta	44.88
4 ounces	Chicken breast (white meat)	187.00
2 Tbsp	Caesar dressing, nonfat	20.00
1 cup	Salad (any veggies)	49.00
		300.88
PM Snack		
15	Almonds	104.04
0.75 cup	Blueberries, raw	60.90
		164.94

Quantity	Description	Calories
Dinner		
0.5 cup	Brown rice, cooked	110.00
2 bunches	Spinach, raw	149.60
1	Turkey burger	419.60
Evening Snack		
1	Low-sugar Fudgsicle	45.00
		45.00
		TOTAL: 1,431.42

Everyday, take:

- Essential oil*
- Nutrients
- 60 to 128 ounces water
- Green tea with afternoon snacks

*My clients take Ultra Essential Oil. It's important for regulating blood sugar; improving digestion; controlling sugar cravings; strengthening and lubricating ligaments, tendons, and joints; maintaining a healthy hormonal balance; and healing and preventing stretch marks and skin problems. Ultra Essential Oil contains rice, soy, sunflower, pumpkin, wheat germ, and olive oils, and it can be bought in the products section of www.ultrafitnutrition.com.

Ultrafit Sample Menu Plan: Day 5

Quantity	Description	Calories
Breakfast		
0.5 cup	Egg Beaters	50.00
1 bunch	Spinach	34.16
1 Tbsp	Essential Oil and Nutrients	120.00
		204.16
AM Snack		
15	Almonds	104.04
1	Apple, medium with peel	81.00
		185.04
Lunch		
0.5 cup	Brown rice, cooked	110.00

1 large (3½" long, 3" diameter)	Pepper, sweet, yellow, raw	50.22
0.5 cup	Tuna, solid white in water	140.00
		300.22
PM Snack		
1	Orange, medium	69.00
3 ounces	Turkey breast (white meat)	114.75
		183.75
Dinner		
1 cup, chopped	Broccoli, raw	24.64
1.5 cups	Ultrafit Nutrition Systems White Lightning Chicken Chili (recipe to follow)	525.00
		549.64
Evening Snack		
1	No-Sugar-Added Fruit Bars	25.00
		25.00
	TOTAL:	**1,447.81**

Everyday, take:

- Essential oil*
- Nutrients
- 60 to 128 ounces water
- Green tea with afternoon snacks

*My clients take Ultra Essential Oil. It's important for regulating blood sugar; improving digestion; controlling sugar cravings; strengthening and lubricating ligaments, tendons, and joints; maintaining a healthy hormonal balance; and healing and preventing stretch marks and skin problems. Ultra Essential Oil contains rice, soy, sunflower, pumpkin, wheat germ, and olive oils, and it can be bought in the products section of www.ultrafitnutrition.com.

Day 5 Recipe

Ultrafit Nutrition Systems White Lightning Chicken Chili

2 tablespoons (30 ml) plus 1½ cups (355 ml) low-fat, low-sodium chicken broth

½ cup (98 g) chopped onion

2 teaspoons minced garlic

2 teaspoons minced jalapeño

1 teaspoon oregano

1 teaspoon cayenne pepper

½ teaspoon ground cumin

Pinch of ground cloves

1 cup (225 g) cooked or canned Great Northern white beans, drained

1 tablespoon (15 ml) lime juice

8 ounces (225 g) skinless, boneless chicken breast, poached and shredded into bite-size pieces

2 tablespoons chopped fresh cilantro or dill

1 tablespoon (5 g) grated Parmesan cheese (nonfat)

1. In a medium soup pot, heat 2 tablespoons (30 ml) broth over medium-high heat. Add the onion and sauté for about 5 minutes, until translucent. Add the garlic, jalapeño, oregano, cayenne, cumin, and cloves. Sauté, stirring occasionally, for about 3 minutes, or until fragrant.

2. Add the beans, lime juice, and remaining 1½ cups (355 ml) of broth and bring to a brisk simmer. Reduce the heat and simmer gently, covered, for 30 minutes. Add the chicken, adjust the seasonings, and heat through.

3. Add the cilantro or dill and stir gently. Ladle into soup bowls, garnish with Parmesan cheese, and serve immediately.

Serving size: 1 cup (255 g), calories: 350, protein: 52 grams, carbs: 30 grams, fat: 6 grams

Ultrafit Sample Menu Plan: Day 6

Quantity	Description	Calories
Breakfast		
2	Egg whites, scrambled/boiled	34.00
0.5 cup	Milk, nonfat	40.00
0.5 cup	Oatmeal, quick, measured uncooked	140.00
1 Tbsp	Essential Oil and Nutrients	120.00
		334.00
AM Snack		
1 container	Protein Shake	230.00
		230.00

Lunch

1 cup, chopped or diced	Broccoli, raw	24.64
0.5 cup	Brown rice, cooked	110.00
4 ounces	Chicken breast (white meat)	187.00
		321.64

PM Snack

0.25 each	Cantaloupe, muskmelon	46.50
0.5 cup	Nonfat cottage cheese	80.00
		126.50

Dinner

1 Tbsp	Fat-free Caesar dressing	10.00
6 ounces	Halibut, broiled	238.50
1 cup	Salad (any veggies)	49.00
1 cup	Yam, baked or boiled	158.00
		455.50
		TOTAL: 1,467.64

Everyday, take:

- Essential oil*
- Nutrients
- 60 to 128 ounces water
- Green tea with afternoon snacks

*My clients take Ultra Essential Oil. It's important for regulating blood sugar; improving digestion; controlling sugar cravings; strengthening and lubricating ligaments, tendons, and joints; maintaining a healthy hormonal balance; and healing and preventing stretch marks and skin problems. Ultra Essential Oil contains rice, soy, sunflower, pumpkin, wheat germ, and olive oils, and it can be bought in the products section of www.ultrafitnutrition.com.

Ultrafit Sample Menu Plan: Day 7

Quantity	Description	Calories
Breakfast		
1 slice	Bread, whole wheat	120.00
1 cubic inch	Cheese, low-fat, Cheddar or Colby	29.41
0.5 cup	Egg Beaters	50.00
1 Tbsp	Essential Oil and Nutrients	120.00
		319.41
AM Snack		
15	Almonds	104.04
6 ounces	Yogurt, light, all flavors	90.00
		194.04
Lunch		
1 cup	Chicken and Asparagus Salad (recipe to follow)	188.00
		188.00
PM Snack		
1.5 cups	Ultrafit Nutrition Systems Protein Smoothie (recipe to follow)	225.00
		225.00
Dinner		
1 cup	Salad (any veggies)	49.00
1	Ultrafit Nutrition Systems Stuffed Pepper with Chicken, Corn, and Cannellini Beans (recipe to follow)	305.00
1 Tbsp	Nonfat Italian dressing	15.00
		369.00
Evening Snack		
1	Low-sugar Fudgsicle	69.00
		69.00
		TOTAL: 1,364.45

Everyday, take:

- Essential oil*
- Nutrients
- 60 to 128 ounces water
- Green tea with afternoon snacks

*My clients take Ultra Essential Oil. It's important for regulating blood sugar; improving digestion; controlling sugar cravings; strengthening and lubricating ligaments, tendons, and joints; maintaining a healthy hormonal balance; and healing and preventing stretch marks and skin problems. Ultra Essential Oil contains rice, soy, sunflower, pumpkin, wheat germ, and olive oils, and it can be bought in the products section of www.ultrafitnutrition.com.

Day 7 Recipes

Chicken and Asparagus Salad

2 $\frac{1}{2}$ cups (335 g) diagonally cut asparagus (1-inch, or 2.5-cm, pieces)

$\frac{1}{2}$ cup (55 g) nonfat mayonnaise

$\frac{1}{2}$ cup (60 g) plain low-fat yogurt

1 teaspoon curry powder

1 teaspoon (5 ml) fresh lemon juice

$\frac{1}{2}$ teaspoon salt

$\frac{1}{8}$ teaspoon ground black pepper

2 cups (220 g) chopped roasted skinless, boneless chicken breasts (about 2 breasts)

$\frac{1}{3}$ cup (50 g) chopped red bell pepper

$\frac{1}{2}$ cup (15 g) chopped fresh flat-leaf parsley

2 tablespoons (15 g) sliced almonds, toasted

1. Steam the asparagus, covered, 2 minutes or until crisp-tender.

2. Combine the mayonnaise, yogurt, curry powder, lemon juice, salt, and black pepper in a large bowl, stirring well with a whisk. Add the asparagus, chicken, bell pepper, parsley, and almonds; toss to coat.

Serving size: 1 cup (225 g) chicken salad mixture; serve with bread or romaine lettuce, calories: 188, protein 25.4 grams, carbs: 10 grams, fat: 5.3 grams

Ultrafit Nutrition Systems Protein Smoothie

½ cup (120 g) plain nonfat yogurt

½ cup (115 g) nonfat cottage cheese

1 cup (250 g) frozen fruit of any kind (strawberries and blueberries make a good smoothie)

1 cup (235 ml) water

Sprinkle of Splenda

1 tablespoon (15 ml) vanilla, for flavor if needed

1 scoop vanilla protein powder (I like Pro Vanilla Protein Powder; any whey, soy, or egg white protein is okay)

1 cup ice

1. Blend all ingredients together in a blender.

Serving size: 2 cups (455 g), calories: 300, protein: 30 grams, carbs: 30 grams, fat: 3 grams

Ultrafit Nutrition Systems Stuffed Peppers with Chicken, Corn, and Cannellini Beans

1 cup (235 ml) water

½ cup (95 g) uncooked brown rice

2 egg whites

8 ounces (225 g) skinless chicken breast, broiled and minced

1 cup (130 g) frozen, thawed corn kernels

1 cup (225 g) low-sodium canned cannellini beans, rinsed and drained

½ cup (125 g) nonfat ricotta

1 clove garlic, minced

½ teaspoon ground black pepper

4 green bell peppers, cut in half horizontally and cored

½ cup (120 ml) nonfat low-sodium chicken broth

½ cup (15 g) chopped fresh parsley

1. Bring the water to a boil in a large saucepan. Stir in the rice; return to a boil, reduce heat, cover, and simmer until rice is just tender, about 20 minutes.

2. Preheat the oven to 450°F (230°C, or gas mark 8).

3. In a large bowl, beat the egg whites. Add the rice, chicken, corn, beans, ricotta, garlic, and black pepper. Stuff the bell pepper halves with this mixture.

4. Arrange in a nonstick baking dish and bake until the peppers are tender, basting with chicken broth, about 40 minutes. Sprinkle with parsley and serve immediately.

Serving size: 1 pepper, calories: 305, protein: 31 grams, carbs: 45 grams, fat: 2 grams

✳ Grocery List for Ultrafit Quick-Start Weight-Loss Menu

Everything that is in your menu, including spices, is on this grocery list. I've grouped similar items together to make it easier for you to shop. I recommend that you look through the list before you go to the grocery store to see what you already have in your pantry, refrigerator, or spice rack. This will save you time and money. You don't have to worry about the brand names—just watch calories to make sure they match up according to your menus.

Fruit

Apples	2
Blueberries	2 cups
Cantaloupe	0.5
Grapefruit	1
Lemon	1
Orange	1
Plum	1
Strawberries	1 cup

Vegetables

Asparagus	4 cups
Basil, fresh	1 tablespoon
Bell peppers, green	4
Bell peppers, red	2
Bell peppers, yellow	2
Broccoli	3 1/2 cups
Cilantro	1 1/2 bunches (8 tablespoons)
Corn, frozen	1 cup
Garlic clove	1
Lettuce	8 cups
Onion	2
Parsley, fresh	1 cup
Spinach	2 bunches
Yam	1

Dry Foods

Almonds	1 bag
Bagel, wheat	1/2 bagel
Bread, wheat	2 slices
Melba toast, wheat	1 box
Oatmeal	1 1/2 cups
Rice, brown	3 cups
Sugar, brown	2 tablespoons
Tortilla, corn	1

Poultry/Meat

Chicken, roasted	1 whole
Chicken breasts	44 ounces
Halibut	6 ounces
Salmon fillets	4 (24 ounces total)
Sea bass fillets	4 (24 ounces total)
Turkey breast	5 ounces
Turkey burger	1

Meal Replacements

Protein bar, low-sugar (Trioplex, Carb Rite)	1
Soy whey protein powder, vanilla	3 scoops

Spices/Seasonings

Black pepper, ground	2 tablespoons
Chili powder	5 tablespoons
Cinnamon	4 tablespoons
Cumin, ground	4 tablespoons
Curry powder	1 tablespoon
Garlic clove, minced	3 tablespoons
Garlic cloves	3
Jalapeño, minced	2 tablespoons
Salt	2 tablespoons
Splenda	20 packets

Juices/Drinks

Green tea	4 bags
Lemon juice	3 tablespoons
Lime juice	1 tablespoon
Pineapple juice	1/2 cup
Water	7 gallons

Frozen Foods

Blueberries	1 cup
Fruit bars, no-sugar	1
Fudgsicles, low-sugar, low-fat	3
Strawberries	1 cup

Canned Foods/Condiments

Cannellini beans, low-sodium, canned	1 can
Chicken broth, low-sodium	4 cups
Chiles, diced	1 (2-ounce) can
Cooking spray, nonfat	1 can
Corn	1 can
Great Northern white beans, canned	1 can
Jelly, low-sugar	1 tablespoon
Olive oil	1 bottle
Parmesan cheese	1 tablespoon
Pineapple preserves	3 tablespoons
Rice vinegar	2 tablespoons
Salad dressing, low-fat	1 bottle
Salsa	1/2 cup
Tuna, canned	1 1/2 cups
Vanilla	2 tablespoons
Worcestershire sauce	2 dashes

Dairy

Cheddar or Colby, low-fat
  3 cubic inches

Cottage cheese, nonfat   2 cups

Cream cheese, nonfat
  1 tablespoon

Egg Beaters   1 cup

Egg whites   13

Feta cheese, reduced-fat
  1 cubic inch

Mayonnaise, nonfat $1/2$ cup

Milk, nonfat   2 cups

Ricotta, nonfat $1/2$ cup

Yogurt, nonfat flavored
  1 (6-ounce) container

Yogurt, nonfat plain $1^{1}/2$ cups

TOP 10 NUTRITIONAL MISTAKES ACTIVE PEOPLE MAKE

1. Skipping breakfast. Not eating breakfast is like asking your car to get you to work without fuel in the tank. It also slows your metabolism. Bottom line: *Eat breakfast!*

2. Not eating before you work out. A preworkout meal consisting of carbs, a little fat, and some protein can help improve endurance and hand-eye coordination.

3. Waiting too long after exercising to eat. After your workout sessions are over, eat a small meal that includes both carbs and protein within two hours. The carbs help replenish muscle glycogen stores, and the protein facilitates the repair of damaged muscle tissue.

4. Replacing meals with energy bars and shakes. Sure, they are convenient, but there is no substitute for healthy whole foods.

5. Eating too much protein and not enough carbs. Whether you are an endurance athlete or bodybuilder (or something in-between), carbs are essential to effective workouts.

6. Trusting the accuracy of dietary supplements labels and claims. Because the supplement industry remains largely unregulated, manufacturers can make unproven and untested claims about their products. Don't fall for the hype and do your homework before putting anything into your body.

7. Not consuming the right amount of calories for the amount of activity you do (i.e., too many or too few). Your caloric intake should be sufficient to support your active lifestyle, but not so abundant that weight control becomes a challenge.

8. Believing that exercise means you can eat whatever you want. Most of us have to learn this lesson the hard way. Whether you exercise a little or a lot, you still need to follow a healthy, balanced diet and watch your portion sizes.

9. Not drinking enough fluids. Dehydration can be a serious problem, especially when you're exercising in the heat. Drinking fluids before, during, and after exercise will help you maintain adequate hydration levels. If you wait to drink when you feel thirsty, you are already dehydrated.

10. Jumping on the latest diet craze. It is tempting to believe that there is some magic pill or formula that will help you achieve that perfect body, but no such magical solution exists. The best thing anyone can do is to stick to the basics and follow a healthy, balanced diet.

Acknowledgments

To Fair Winds Press: Thanks to Holly, Wendy, and crew for asking me to write this book. Thanks again to Rosalind for being so accommodating by flying to San Diego for my second photo shoot so I could be with my family. It was so much fun having you and Allan spend time with my family at dinner. To Allan: Even though you are a smart butt, I love ya! I think that great photography truly makes a book and your photos are beautiful.

To my *Ultrafit* book contributors: First, I want to thank Hannah Sansone for her contribution to this book. I love how you understand me and know how to snap me out of a writing block at any time. Without you, I would never get anything done.

Second, I would like to thank Trish Vasper, my Ultrafit general manager, for managing my company so I can work on projects like this book. I have all the confidence in the world in you, and I am so thankful to have someone so dedicated to Ultrafit and such a loyal employee! I love you! Thanks to Dale Webber for your help with the photo shoot. You are a beautiful person inside and out!

Thanks to Neil Mallinson for your input on my exercises and for being honest about an exercise that I made up that didn't quite make sense.

Now to my husband Mike: The reason I am where I am today is because of you. Your constant support in all my business endeavors gives me the confidence and support I need to succeed. I feel so blessed to have you in my life and so thankful for your love and for being the best dad to our little girls.

Next, to my two babies, Jaden and Kendall: I don't remember life without you. You have changed who I am and how I look at life.

To my parents: Thanks to my mom and dad, Mona and Ken, for all your support. You gave me the confidence to follow my passion and never look back!

To Sharon and Jim Hill: You two are like my parents. Your love and support is tremendous.

To my sisters: Kristin and Amy, thank you for all you do for me, your love and friendship means the world to me!

To my Ultrafit staff: To Jessica, my first consultant, Brooke, Neil, Anna, Marjorie, Jess, Carolyn, Shellie, Erica, Heather, Mandy, Lori, Matt, Suzanne, and Kirsten. Thank you for all your hard work for Ultrafit!

Thanks to Frogs Club One, The Monday Group, Jeff Kotterman, and NASN!

To Hample Construction: Thanks, Danny and Jackie Hample, for allowing us to shoot the photos for this book and my *Ultrafit* book in your beautiful homes that you build. You can never stop building homes! What would I do without them? Ha!

To my sponsor Nike: Thanks so much, Nike, for believing in me and for always supplying my apparel and shoes. Shane, you rock!

To my sponsor Oakley and Al Janc: Thanks, Oakley and Al Janc, for your awesome sunglasses and support!

To my friends: To my friends who make my life more balanced—Nikki, Cindy, Susan, Misha, Kersten, Nicole, Jessica, Margo, Jen, and my NBF Kim. It's five o'clock somewhere, isn't it?

To my television friends: KUSI News—Susan Lennon, Dan Plant, Alyson, Libby, and everyone at the station who makes me feel so at home for my weekly segment.

And last but not at all least, to the people who work so hard to make me look good! Special thanks Nicole Howard, and my friends at Salon Radius, David, Abbey, Courtney, and Amanda.

✳ Resources, Web sites, and Recommended Reading

American Association of Neurological Surgeons,
www.neurosurgerytoday.org

American Council on Exercise (ACE),
www.acefitness.org

BioForce Golf, from Sean M. Cochran,
www.bioforcegolf.com

Body Building for You,
www.Bodybuildingforyou.com

Cleveland Clinic, www.clevelandclinic.org

Fit 365, www.getfit365.com

Frogs Fitness Clubs, www.Frogsfitness.com

Georgia State University, The Exercise and
Physical Fitness Page (strength-training tips,
including illustrations),
http://www.gsu.edu/~wwwfit/strength.html

Mayo Clinic, www.mayoclinic.com

**National Institute of Neurological Disorders
and Stroke,** www.ninds.nih.gov

Optimum Life (holistic fitness and stress
management), http://optimumlife.co.nz

Partners in Beauty, www.partnersinbeauty.com.

The Physician and Sportsmedicine,
http://www.physsportsmed.com/issues/1998/02feb/s
tamford.htm

Sports Performance Group,
http://www.woodspg.com/

Ultrafit Nutrition Systems, www.Ultrafitnutrition.com

Chu, Donald A. *Explosive Power and Strength.*
Champaign, IL: Human Kinetics, 1996.

Daniels, D. *Pilates Perfect: The Complete Guide to
Pilates Exercise at Home.* Long Island City, NY: A
Healthy Living Book, 2003, 130–196.

Fiscella, Catherine. "Help for Low Back Pain." IDEA
Fitness Journal, September 2005, 34.

Gillies, Elizabeth. *101 Ways to Work Out on the Ball,*
Gloucester, MA: Fair Winds Press, 2004

Journal of Clinical Endocrinology and Metabolism vol.
81, 1312–17. Peterson, MD, MR Rhea, and BA
Alvar, "Maximizing Strength Development in
Athletes."

Journal of Strength and Conditioning 18(4): 723–29,
2004. Starr, Bill. "The Value of Warming Up and
Stretching," www.EricsGym.com.

ACSM Fitness Book. Indianapolis, IN: American College
of Sports Medicine, 1992.

Aerobics and Fitness Association of America. *Fitness
Theory and Practice.* 2nd ed., ed. Peg Jordan.
Stoughton, MA: Reebok University Press, 1997.

Alman, Brian. *Keep It Off.* New York: Plume, 2004.

Karter, Karon. *Pilates Lite.* Gloucester, MA: Fair Winds
Press, 2004.

Kosich, Daniel. *Get Real.* IDEA, 1995.

Kraus, Barbara. *Calories and Carbohydrates.* 8th ed.
New York: Penguin Group, 1988.

Lifestyle and Weight Management Consultant Manual.
Ed. Richard T. Cotton and Christine J. Ekeroth.
San Diego, CA: American Council on Exercise
(ACE), 1996.

National Strength and Conditioning Association.
Essentials of Strength Training and Conditioning.
Ed. Thomas R. Baechle and Roger W. Early.
Champaign, IL: Human Kinetics, 2000.

Radcliffe, James C., and Robert C. Farentinos.
High-Powered Plyometrics. Champaign, IL:
Human Kinetics, 1999.

Rinzler, Carol Ann. *Nutrition for Dummies.* 3rd ed.
Indianapolis, IN: Wiley Publishing, 2004.

Twining, Glenda, with Arnold Wayne Jones. *Yoga Fights
Flab.* Gloucester, MA: Fair Winds Press, 2004.

Twining, Glenda, with Mark Seal. *Yoga Turns Back the
Clock.* Gloucester, MA: Fair Winds Press, 2003.

Webb, Tamilee, with Cheryl Fenton. *Defy Gravity
Workout.* Gloucester, MA: Fair Winds Press, 2005.

About the Author

Today a celebrated nutrition and fitness guru, **Cindy Whitmarsh** is the owner of Ultrafit Nutrition Systems, a fitness and nutrition consulting business she runs out of Four Frogs Club One Health Clubs in Southern California and is expanding to clubs throughout the state. Cindy is an NASN-licensed sports nutritionist and fitness instructor. She is the creator of the *Ultrafit Fat-Burning Workout* video and starred in the *10-Minute Solution, Target Toning* video. She is the author of the books *Ultrafit: Challenging Workouts, Amazing Results,* and *Ultrafit Cooking*. Cindy is a regular contributor to numerous fitness and nutrition publications, as well as local radio and television programs. She also writes nutrition and fitness programs for fitness videos, other fitness experts, and Web sites. Creator of her own annual fitness competition, "The Ms. Ultrafit Competition," Cindy also cohosts a national infomercial for Power Reactor Fitness and is the health and fitness reporter for KUSI Television in San Diego, California. She also hosted her own radio show called "The Weight Loss Hour," cohosted by Dr. Brian Alman. Cindy's latest project is a program for kids called "Ultrafit Kids." She is working on a fitness video for kids, Web site, protein shake, protein bar, and much more.

Her high-profile clientele includes numerous television personalities, radio DJs, and professional athletes, including her husband, pro beach volleyball player Mike Whitmarsh. Cindy and Mike have two baby girls. Cindy is passionate about health, wellness, and longevity, and she loves to share her experience and results with the world.

Also from Fair Winds

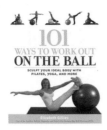

101 WAYS TO WORK OUT ON THE BALL
By Elizabeth Gillies
ISBN-13: 978-1-59233-084-3
ISBN-10: 1-59233-084-3
$19.95/£12.99/$27.95
Paperback; 176 pages
Available wherever books are sold

Everyone loves the workout ball! It can help with weight training, Pilates, yoga, and even cardio and stretching moves. *101 Ways to Work Out on the Ball* gives you exercises that will strengthen, lengthen, tone, and stretch your body like no other form of exercise can. The moves will work for beginners, intermediate, and advanced exercisers; some even require weights to sculpt your arms and legs while strengthening your core.

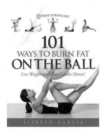

101 WAYS TO BURN FAT ON THE BALL
By Lizbeth Garcia
ISBN-13: 978-1-59233-207-6
ISBN-10: 1-59233-207-2
$19.95/£12.99/$27.95 CAN
Paperback; 192 pages
Available wherever books are sold.

Incorporating the ball into your heart-pounding cardio routines and your strengthening and toning sessions is a lot easier than you think! Inside, you'll find 101 illustrated moves and step-by-step instructions demonstrating how to use your fitness ball to boost your metabolism, build muscle, and lose weight. Whether you've been using the ball in your workouts for years or you're a ball beginner, you'll discover that these simple and effective exercises are the sparks you need to re-energize your workouts and finally get the results you've been waiting for.

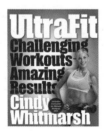

ULTRAFIT
By Cindy Whitmarsh
ISBN-13: 978-1-59233-175-8
ISBN-10: 1-59233-175-0
$19.95/£12.99/$27.95 CAN
Paperback; 192 pages
Available wherever books are sold.

Let fitness expert Cindy Whitmarsh challenge your conventional workout ways and what you thought were good eating habits to help you achieve new heights of fitness success! *Ultrafit* is an innovative exercise and nutrition program built for people of all ages and fitness levels. The program consists of three different stages, allowing you to jump right in at your current ability level and use the same routines and nutrition advice that Olympians and professional athletes have been using for years to crank up their games a notch. A bonus DVD is also included, featuring a 20-minute workout. This workout blast, yoga stretch, and cooldown stretch allows you to get the energizing routine you need—whenever you need it.